Grumpy & Me

From 9-to-5 to 24/7:
The Unofficial Guide to
Marriage in Retirement

By Meg Marlow
2025

This trade paperback is published by Grumpy's Guild.

Cataloging Information
ISBN: 978-1-0369-6753-6
Credits
Editor: Nicci Robinson
Cover Design: Nicci Robinson
Illustrations: KC Lylark
Production Design: Global Wordsmiths

Acknowledgements

I'd like to thank my husband, Michael, not only for his support, but also for providing a constant source of material with his good humour. I'd be lost without him but kindly don't tell him that.

Thank you to my readers for their loyalty and belief that I *did* have a book in me, and especially Olwyn Vissenga, who badgered me to start my blog way back in 2016. Ta muchly, you lovely bunch.

And of course, to Nicci Robinson of Global Wordsmiths. Her patience and advice have been amazing.

Dedication

For my mam.
She may have had nothing,
but she gave me everything.

A bit about Grumpy & Me

We met way back in 1969 at a cousin's wedding. I was seventeen years old and new to the Civil Service, having fallen into the role when my dad insisted it was a good job for a woman. Michael was twenty-one and in the same paratroopers' regiment as the groom.

There are some things you can, in my opinion, never go back on. Your word. And cutting your fringe.

Which is how we remain married after almost fifty-five years. We did much better than the bride and groom, who were divorced within five years. If you look closely, you can still see the para in Michael's soul. And my dad was right: my job allowed me to work and raise our three daughters.

Relationships are rarely a bed of roses. They're more likely to be a bed of porcupines, which is how you develop a thick skin in order to survive. We've had good times, bad times, and times that cutting each other's livers out came very close. There's no one I'd trust more to slice mine out.

We settled down in a suburb of my home town, Newcastle, and we had our first daughter in 1972, a second in 1974, and a third followed in 1991. You can see we've never really been planners. In 2011, we migrated south to Cheshire to join our daughters.

My heart still belongs to Newcastle, but Cheshire has been good to us.

Me

I'M NOT A demonstrable sentimentalist. I don't choose to wear my heart on my sleeve. I much prefer it tucked away safely where I can't lose it. Next to my stiff upper lip, which is easily stiffened further by over-sugary sweetness.

I blame my mam, who rubbed everything better with briskness. And a damp hanky.

I find my people when I scratch the surface and unearth their witty sarcasm. Nice folk worry me; they're hiding something. I much prefer the blunt bread knife people. They'll butter my bread nicely and not slather it in too much jam.

If Grumpy had a nice wife, he wouldn't know what to do with himself. He needs someone who's a challenge. I know this to be true because I told him so.

I like to think that I'm very rarely shocked by what

I'm told. I'd have to rethink that statement if I ever met a serial killer, of course. Although, rudeness rankles my cankles no end. It shouldn't come as a surprise that if you're a twat, I'll call you one. But as Mr God's son said, "Let him without a socially unacceptable issue cast the first Twitter." Well, he would've done if they'd ever done a remake of the Bible. You know, like they do with classic films...which are never as good as the original.

Where was I? Oh, yes, mid-pontification.

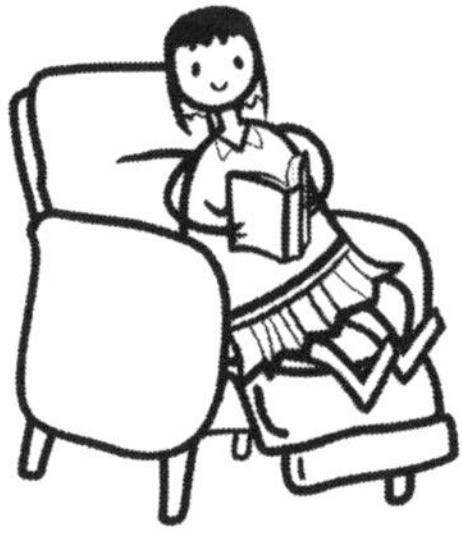

What I'm trying to say is that I write to amuse you and me. I write to share this strange thing called old age. I write because it clears my mind. Grumpy gives no figs that I'm writing about him too. Indeed he will often quip, "There's one for your blog" when he cocks something up. For which I'm eternally grateful.

I know that, occasionally, I may sound ungrateful for what I have, which, after years of training, is a jolly decent spouse. Or I don't realise that one day, I may be left on my own. But just like my mam scrubbed away with love and told me that we're always more viciously tongued with the ones we love the most, my mantra with my daughters is always "pull yourself together." We all paint love in different ways and, like art, some folk won't appreciate your style, but your people will. So paint for *them*.

The Vintage Model

CONGRATULATIONS! YOU ARE now the proud owner of a vintage body. Please read the following instructions to ensure you keep it running smoothly:

- The temperature control may malfunction. We suggest you purchase clothing that will slip on, over or under—quickly.
- Buttons are not your friend, be they on clothing or inanimate objects, such as the TV remote. Or your husband. Do *not* attempt to push them. It's very easy to trigger crossed wires that will mean a loss of sound over several days.
- Please keep upright to avoid unnecessary breakages.
- Replacement parts are difficult to come by. There may be a few languishing in the corridors of the NHS. But there will be a need to jump through hoops to attain a new hip or knee, for

instance. Kindly refer to the above rule.

- Vintage models eventually lapse and run on mono, not stereo, sound. There may be static interference. This is normal. We suggest closing the lounge doors so the husband's mutterings are greatly reduced.
- Do not immerse fully in water. It takes longer than expected to dry out, and difficult to reach crevices could become susceptible to fungus.
- Your model will not always compute as quickly as newer models. However, its power of reasoning increases intensely. There's a 99% chance it will stubbornly refuse to change course.
- Unlike recent models, they do not need to announce to all and sundry when the sun comes up.
- It is usual to hear rogue noises from an unexpected item in the bagging area when attempting to lift a bag of groceries that has cost 50% of your State Pension.
- Aforementioned noises are not to be confused with actual body noises. Usually, these will be ball and socket joint-related. This is to be expected. You've run out of oil. Unlike Kuwait.

To balance this out, you will unearth a new supply of natural gas, pockets of which will escape when you least expect it.

- Do not fiddle with any knobs. They will not turn anything on.
- Batteries go flatter quicker. Recharge regularly. In an emergency, Kit Kats will provide an instant boost.
- Their own counsel is kept safe and secure at all times.
- Vintage models will not tolerate severe weather. Unlike modern models, they will not increase alcohol levels to overcome the heat or cold, they will instead go for cotton or woollen garments. And tea.
- They will not use alcohol for recreational use. It will be purely medicinal—and flavoured.
- These models close down from social intercourse at 6:59 p.m. precisely.
- We suggest you take great care of these vintage models. They are irreplaceable.

Growing Up

WHEN I WAS a young girl, I thought I would always be so. The concept of ageing never darkened the doorstep of my mind.

My aged aunties had an annoying habit of calling me any family name, various dog names, the pet cats, and twice the budgies. Any name except my own.

When they repeated the same stories as if they were telling them for the first time, I rolled my eyes.

The constant hunt for glasses, a shilling for the meter, the whispered command to hide from the tick man behind the sofa, and any tale that began "When we were young" were the stuff of *old people*. The wireless got ever louder as the years rolled by.

I loved the old dears.

Dressed in sensible stout shoes, always with a clean pinny pulled around their expanding waistlines and topped off with a knitted cardigan. The lines of laughter and sorrow were etched in their faces in equal amounts. They smelled of family, safety, and warmth.

There was nothing better than a Saturday afternoon at my granny's in Byker, listening to them gossip. Or watching any one of them with a poss tub and hot bubbling water, washing on a Monday morning. And only ever on Monday, with the scent of Omo filling the air.

I started school. They looked the same.

I left school. They looked the same.

I took a job at the "Ministry," earning seven shillings a week. They looked the same.

As my skirts got shorter and my ambitions higher, they tutted louder. As my snakeskin boots rolled up my legs, they sniggered at modern day fashion and the very idea of wearing pretend python. When I donned my bottle green PVC mac, they almost swallowed their dentures in mirth. They looked the same.

What did they know, with their sensible bras and corsets?

I was still Jean, Eleanor, Hilary, Bobby, Frankie, Margaret, Bluey, Fifi, George, or Bob to them.

Then one by one, they left my life.

Grumpy & Me

I thought they'd always be there: Aunty Nellie making apple pies; Aunty Bella with her acidic tongue more tart than the cooking apples; Aunty Lizzie sneaking off to the bookies. And me mam? Well, she would always be there.

Except she wasn't.

They weren't.

And now it's my turn. Tag, I'm it.

Bastarding old age has done what it does best. I'm one of the older generation, who the younger generation think are quite bonkers. Slightly Lady Gaga. Sick. Cute. I've always looked the same age to them. I've never been young.

I'm fucked if I can recall their names. Yesterday, I lost my bank card. It'll soon be my marbles.

Harriet, Dominic, Arabella, Christian, or Camilla... They're still thinking they'll never age.

Poetry Without Motion

It is nine thirty in the morning,
I must now make a start.
I need to get the hoover out,
stop being a lazy tart,
I shall dust, and sweep, and tidy,
The house will soon begin to glow.
And with my trusty tin of Pledge, a-dusting I will go
I'll check my phone before I start
That took an hour or so,
And then I mentally tick myself off,
"Get up you sloth and go."

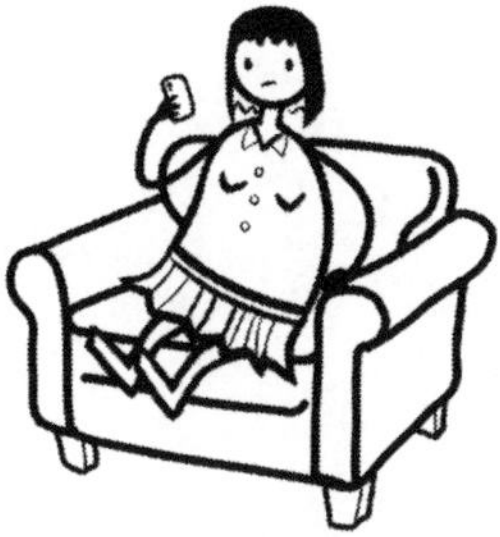

But I glimpse a crossword empty
In my *Take A Break*,
I cannot leave that undone
So another half hour I take,
By now it is eleven
And time to make a brew,
I shall also have a biscuit,
Oh fuck it, I'll take two.

Ready, steady, here I go,
my pinny's tied on tight.
In half an hour, I will be done,
the house all clean and bright.
I shall pick up and put some things away
before I wash the floor.
But once more get distracted
by the postman at the door.
Oh, joy! Oh, bliss! Why look at this!
My magazine has come,
And before I even know it,
I am sat down on my bum.

The clock chimes two,
oh, deary me,

Grumpy & Me

I have not yet begun.
What was it I was doing?
What should I have begun?
My polish and my cloth and my vacuum look and stare
While I look around the house from the comfort of my chair.
Oh, shite with this, I whisper, what was it Scarlett said?
"Tomorrow is another day."
I shall clean it then instead.

Better Bit of Butter

GRUMPY (ON OPENING the fridge, standing there in his underpants, and after a good chill): "Where's the butter?"

Me: "I don't know. Where *is* the butter?"

"It's not here!"

"Where?"

"Here! In the butter space!"

"Indeed, the empty butter space. For there is no butter!"

There may be no butter, but I can still see a knob.

I was away at the weekend. On my departure, Grumpy attempted his bestest sad face. It's a shite sad face, because it looks very much like a great big cheesy, upturned mouth, happy face. I could read in his eyes the joy of not shaving, leaving the toilet seat up, sleeping in the shade in the garden on a lounger, a mid-afternoon beer...or three. Followed by peeing on the peonies.

Nowhere in Grumpy's plans was a visit to the shops. Nor would he awaken the vacuum. He was on a restation.

Tough titties.

In retirement, we are both equal. Grumpy has the exact same ability as me to see the butter rations were low. In the absence of a Butter Fairy, he would need to shop for more.

It's not unusual to run out of things. An empty wrapper is usually the clue. Except for those people who place empty packets back on the shelf. And we *all* know one of those, don't we, ladies? Because empty packets, toilet rolls, and bottles are *far* too heavy to hold whilst pressing a pedal bin into action.

I held my ground. I knew *he* knew *I* knew he should have collected more butter supplies instead of waiting for my return in the hopes that I would be packing a pound of butter in my suitcase.

I wasn't.

Grumpy harrumphed and went to the shop. And returned with three packs of tomatoes and a hot sausage sandwich.

Luckily for him, I was already out. On the way home,

I called at the shop too. I also rang him to check if we needed anything.

Grumpy: "Erm, nope. Nil. Nothing. I did go to the shops too, you know?"

Me: "Sure??"

"Pffft!"

And down the phone goes. And the pretty butterflies dance in the space in his head where there almost used to be a brain.

This morning, at two minutes before eight of the clock, Grumpy returns to the bedroom to ask where the butter is. I tell him that as far as I know, it's still in the cow called Daisy. In a field in France. In the sun.

His final bovine remark leaves him reeling after a glance on the head from my well-aimed, half-full plastic water bottle. And if I *was* a cow, I would be called Marigold.

Betty may have bought a bit of butter, but dopey Grumpy didn't...

And he could really use some for that nasty bump on his head.

Do You Remember When Going to Bed Was Fun?

WHEN YOU WOULD drop into it wearily, close your eyes, and wake up, fully refreshed? Or when sleep was the last thing on your mind as you headed for the boudoir? Wasn't life grand?

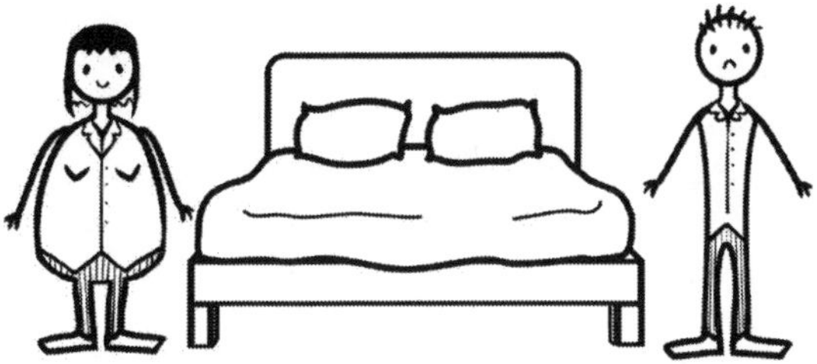

And then, as you balance on the precipice of retirement:

You will treat yourself to a mattress costing more than your first second-hand car to help you to sleep better. You won't. Because the second your eyelids droop at 11:30 of the p.m, your bladder remembers the .00035ml of piss stored in the bilge that needs to be expelled...approximately every two hours. Unless you were silly enough to enjoy an alcoholic nightcap. In which case, that time scale is reduced to every forty-seven minutes. In between, you will hear the warthog next to you achieve a crescendo of snoring, broken only by the phut, phut, phut of light sleep REM that makes you consider put, put, putting them out of their misery with the ridiculously priced memory foam pillow you're hugging.

Lost in thought, you will be struck by pain: in your hips, shoulder, wrists, the gristly bit of your ear, knuckle, and knees. And slaver that has welded the side of your face to the duvet. Plus hunger pains. You're fortunate you ate a sneaky custard cream before disrobing, the crumbs of which are gathered under your right boob. Champion.

You will lie in the dark and count the threads on your Egyptian cotton sheets. Except you're now thirsty. You refuse to budge. And slip into a light sleep where you dream of an oasis in the Gobi Desert. Your eyes flick open. You fret if you locked the back door, closed the window in the bathroom. Did you check the gas rings?

Grumpy & Me

Put the cat out? Does Donald Trump wear a wig?

You really need to pee. And your tongue is stuck to the roof of your mouth.

Your concentration becomes clearer when you realise you have encountered a rogue limb splayed across your torso. You do a recount. It's definitely not your own. In disgust, you lob it like a hand grenade at your companion. They swipe it upward then downwards towards their nether regions, where they scratch with such relish that you decide to take this opportunity to have your third pee of the night. So far.

It is 2:27 a.m. Despite knowing every inch of the bedroom, you will twat your bunion on the bedpost. On both the outward and inward journey. To welcome you back, your companion farts, a clawing stench that bores into your very soul. Unrepentant, you use their own dentures from the bedside cabinet to bite their arse.

It's no good now; sleep evades you. You've put various parts of your body in and out of the bed so much that you've played a full solo range of the "Hokey Cokey." Your nightwear is wedged under your third chin in a strangle hold, but somehow, the residue is being eaten by your vulva.

With one more final toss onto your back you will make a mental to do list for tomorrow. You are confident you will remember it. You won't.

By 5:17 a.m., you will give in and get up. Then you'll make a cup of tea, sit down, and fall fast asleep upright in your HSL chair.

Give Us a Clue

OH, SHIRLEY, OH, Deborah, oh, Julie, oh, Jane, I forget your name. I forget your name...

Jennifer, Alison, Phillipa, Sue, Deborah, Annabel too. I forget your name...

"Mum!"

"I know. I know. Give me a second. Or a clue..."

Children. So sodding sensitive. It's not like you *deliberately* don't remember their name. You chose it, probably because you liked it. But now, it could be anything. Sometimes I think, "What do they look like?" as I'm rummaging through the piles of crap covered in dust that languish unused in my brain for the file marked, "Baby Names I Really Like. Version 3."

"Norman." Annoyed and Narked Norman. That makes me snigger and gets them more Agitated Agatha. It's okay for them. I'm just Mum.

"MUMMMMMMM!"

It's not just names. I drive. I have no recollection of driving. I shop—for the same thing. I currently have thirteen tins of tuna, twenty tins of chopped tomatoes, six jars of lemon curd, and enough toilet rolls to build Trump's wall... Well, they're used to shite. I write. *An leav od lette off a wor*. My once neat handwriting looks like a spider with three broken legs has fallen into a vat of ink and then hobbled all over my paper.

I wear things inside out. That's not so bad. People think I'm twenty-six. I wear things tucked into my knickers.

The other day, I nipped into the corner shop for wine and chocolate. Grasping the wine to my chest, I paid for the chocolate. And left, only remembering that I'd inadvertently shoplifted as I put the car into first gear and ended up reversing.

I also tell the same story. On loop. Then I forget to pass on vital messages, since those apparently drop straight into the rubbish bin of my brain. Sometimes, I wish I could clear my own head's cache, though not so much the cookies. I like food.

Then there is the loss of a word. It fucks right off mid-sentence. So you try to describe the word for potato masher to a piss-taking husband. You look like you're miming having a stroke. He stops laughing when you retrieve the bastard from the cupboard and menacingly go in for "creamy, yet firm" on his head.

I find spectacles in the fridge. Biscuits in the freezer. And I once tried to pay for my weekly shopping with my senior railcard. Oh, how the young cashier laughed and laughed. Miserable fucker just stood there looking like I'd passed her warm dog shit without a poo bag.

Folk say that their mind wanders. Mine takes itself off to the Seychelles for an all-inclusive holiday and refuses to take calls.

I've heard crosswords help train your brain. My brain hides all the Biros in advance.

Yet strangely, as my mind mists over like a windscreen on a cold day regarding recent events, it sparkles like it's been rinsed with Windolene on days gone by. I can recall every neighbour, aunty, uncle, dog, bus number, song, and the taste of proper Black Jacks from circa 1961.

The fact that I write everything down in a notebook should help...

Except I can't remember where I put it.

Going of the Out

AND JUST LIKE that, Mr Grumpy has made me into a fibber. Well, since meeting him, he's also made me a blasphemer, neurotic, an alcoholic (reformed), and rather stout from overfeeding (unreformed, but trying), so I should have seen it coming.

We have been out.

Twice. Three times, if you include a browse in M&S for some custard tarts after an eye test. I could see them *much* better than the bottom line of the Snellen Chart. I wondered if I'd accidentally loaned him the wrong medication, because we've now entered that dark realm of saving and trading medication. We're at the time of life when we simply don't care. We're no longer knocking on heaven's door; we've reached the age where we've had keys cut. I mean, we're not trading Molly on street corners. And the closest we get to weed is the dandelions in the garden.

Just a few painkillers, the odd statin, and out of date ointments. Ointments are the most contrary. With fading eyesight, it's difficult to read if they're for your arse or your elbow. If you sniff it and your eyes water, that's the haemorrhoid cream.

We only trade with each other to get us through to the next prescription, because our poor chemist can't keep up with the drug habits of our village's ageing population. Three have already made a run for it and started working for a Mexican cartel in Salford. Apparently, they work shorter days selling just the one product. If any customers complain, they're simply shot. Plus, they get all the enchiladas they can eat for lunch, whilst they never had time to eat a healthy protein bar at our branch of Boots. You can see the attraction.

But I do take care when I'm dealing. You know, the same dosage and still in date...roughly. Although, I'll freely admit that I have once accidentally mixed up fungal cream with cold sore cream. I should have noticed the tubes are completely different sizes. In my defence, at least I didn't hand him the Deep Heat.

So, sorry, I'm off-piste. Oh, and if I have to add "Don't try this at home" to the above paragraph, you're reading the wrong book.

Yes, anyway. This week, following my complaints about being boring, there's been a revolution. We've been out to visit a field full of fat-faced, cheery sunflowers dancing in the breeze. Two pensioners and sixtytwelvehundred holidaying Gusset Gremlins, off school for the summer. All of us were gabbling in delight until suddenly, the sunflowers, weary of our marauding, began, in Grumpy's words, "Sticking the nut" on us like big, glowing, jaundiced thugs.

Believe me when I tell you, when a sunflower nuts you, you know about it. Obviously, the fresh air made us giddy (unless I'd cocked the meds up again), because we enjoyed ourselves despite the bruises.

We Are Watching Each Other Grow Old

UP UNTIL RETIREMENT, work, family, life, and living acted as a distraction.

The Pausing of the Men will have the same effect as crunching your car into a brick wall for many marriages. You didn't see it coming. You have no idea how long recovery will take. And for the male, he's probably wondering if it's an appropriate time to part-exchange for a newer model. My advice is to just stick with what you know. If you get a new one that has improved performance, a gleaming chassis, and not much going on under the bonnet, you're going to have to get used to managing it, right smack-bang during your own mid-life crisis. Concentrate on watching your waistline grow as your hair stops...on your head yet grows with increased velocity in your ears, your eyebrows, and from your nasal passages. And while it's true that menopause makes the woman in your life forget, they *never* forgive.

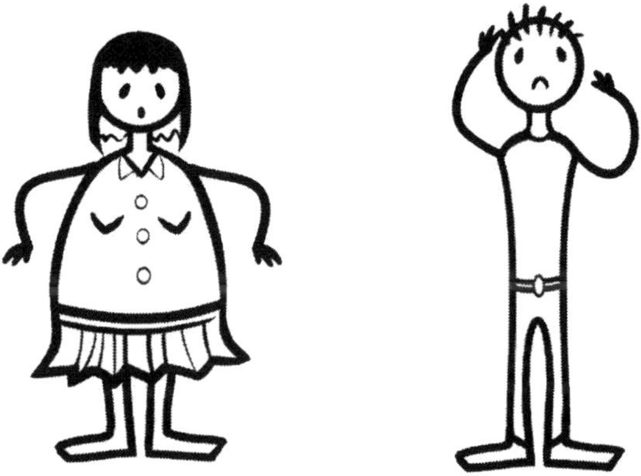

Young Grumpy actually wasn't grumpy at all. He was agile as a cat and had a love for heights. Yet, watching him taking tiles off a shed roof recently was quite nerve-racking. His sure-footedness has left him. He may occasionally smell like an old mountain goat, but he no longer has their agility.

The other day, I sat clutching my Maltesers close to my chest, when one little bugger was lost in transit between my fat fingers and delicate rosebud mouth. It rolled under the sofa. I leave none of my team behind. I got down on the floor to retrieve it and deposited it into my gullet. Before finding that, for the life of me, I couldn't get back up. My bones creaked and popped but wouldn't allow me to do the simple act of standing up. Bastards.

Our hair has changed. We are both grey and follically challenged. Grumpy has fluffy, downy hair. My hair is thinning. My body may not concede and thin down, but my hair could win the "Slimmer of the Year" award from Weight Watchers...for the last seven years in a row.

Suddenly, you have all the time in the world to see youth slipping away, and in its absence, the map of your partner's face changes. The familiarity is still there. The warmth is still there. And the eyes still glow with mischief. But a lot is lost to the years behind those wrinkles. My lipstick bleeds on my fraying lips, so much so, it needs a blood transfusion.

When I read that male urine keeps cats from crapping on your gravel, I gave Grumpy an empty J2O bottle and asked him to provide the goods. His response was to suggest an empty Vicks jar would suffice. Which he would half-fill every hour, on the hour, and three times in ten minutes before we should be leaving the house to go shopping.

We have a bigger supply of drugs between us than a Mexican Cartel. Drugs that make us do. Drugs that make us don't. Although I will not have a Werther's Original in my house. There is no bigger sign of ageing than having a bowl of them sat next to your sofa. Fuck that. I already wear sensible shoes, because kitten heels left me walking like Dick Emery at the recent wedding. Grumpy is never happier than sat in his cardigan and slippers. He also hides Werther's Originals in his car.

When we declare, "Words fail me," it is the truth.

It Should Come with a Warning

Us ladies have three times in our life when circumstances will be beyond our control. Motherhood. Menopause. Retirement. All three will fuck you up and leave you with mental scars. And remove part of your soul. Today, we shall be looking at the final chapter, which is so very much akin to the first.

The middle chapter is yours, and yours alone.

For many years, you dream of retirement. A life on the ocean waves. Ladies Who Luncheon. Afternoon matinees—which is champion, until the partner joins you. The partner whom, despite living under the same roof for several decades, you have spent no more than two weeks alone with since saying. "I do." Before you know it, retirement with your husband is like being a new mum.

Congratulations! You have both retired.

You're now in sole charge of a strange being with a crinkly face that needs feeding and entertaining, and will wake you in the dead of night for no particular reason, other than he wants to know if you're awake since he is. Sleep is denied him until the nanosecond you're wide awake, and then he's immediately snoring like a pot-bellied Vietnamese pig. In appreciation of you being right there with him, he will deliver a rancid fart as a token of love.

You're sure things will get better. It's all a big change. The face looks familiar, but there's a lot more to it than you've ever seen before. You don't know if you're ready for it. You quite liked the independent you, surrounded by colleagues who, just a few weeks hence, sent you cards denoting "Happy Retirement!" and "We will miss you!" You wonder if you should've worked a tad longer. A much cheaper, more nubile, and IT literate twenty-five-year-old is now sitting in your very chair. At your desk. And her name has already replaced yours in the tea club.

It is just you and the husband. 24/7.

Expect to make regular visits to the doctor. For him, not you. Something will always be getting stuck where it should not get stuck. Occasionally, you may be responsible. He will start tinkering with things, sticking chubby little fingers into sockets and knocking things together. He is to DIY what George Clarke is to big spaces: a void. He will take up new hobbies faster than Katie *Tut-Tut* Price picks up new beaus, hobbies that involve trips to B&Q. And large tools (the biggest being the one paying).

Never, ever have your tits been gotten on so much. Even when you were actually breastfeeding. Nothing will prepare you for the questions:

"What are you doing?"

"Why?"

"What's to eat?"

"Why do I have to get washed?"

"Why do I have to go?"

"What are you doing now?"

Nothing will prepare you for the tantrums:

"I am not wearing that!"

"I am *not* eating that!"

"You can't make me!"

"I do not like him/her/them/that/this programme/ you!"

"I am dying! It's not a cold!"

"You were nicer when you had hormones!"

Nothing will prepare you for the interfering:

"Not like that. Like this"

"You don't want to be doing that"

"Leave that to me"

"It would be better if..."

"I think you/we should..."

"I *know* what I'm doing"

You wonder if those homicidal urges you're having are normal. Is there not a clause for diminished responsibility?

Do not compare yourself to other couples who take to retirement like a duck to water. They are simply twats. Never believe social media photos showing George and Betty *#soblessedinCapeVerde* while you're on a day trip to Llandudno. In the rain. With soggy sandwiches. Looking for the toilets. For him, not you.

Do remember to give yourself time to adjust to your new life. Take any help offered. Let the family step in and take over caring. For a week. Or six, so you can bugger off to Benidorm and drink cocktails at two p.m. Alone.

Do *not* expect them to listen to you unless it involves food, the TV remote, or the fact you're going out. If you do, by some chance, let them overhear your plans for a night out with friends, they will do their utmost to stop you from leaving, going so far as to swallow the front door key.

The house is no longer quiet. The house is no longer clean. And there is always some unidentified object waiting for you down the toilet.

You will never exit the house in anything less than three quarters of an hour after the scheduled departure time. This will be down to a lost shoe; the need to pee; them needing a snack; a minor tantrum about wanting to watch the end of something; or it's raining and they don't like getting their hair wet.

Do *not* be fooled and offer them the option to stay behind. You might as well drop them off at social services, you heartless bitch.

Nobody warned you about this.

Just when you've come close to packing a suitcase, you glimpse them fast asleep in bed...sleeping like an angel. And you forgive them all the misdemeanours of the day. Until they start to aggravate you anew tomorrow.

"Tell Me Where It Is!"

ME: "NO!"

Grumpy: "I'm getting annoyed!"

"Makes a change from being miserable."

"Woman, are you looking to vex me!"

"Nope!"

"You're being very childish."

"Yep."

"I just need it for a few minutes."

"Well, you should have got yourself one. This one is mine. Which means it's not yours. And as owner, I'm not willing to lend it to you. Because you're like a navvy. No."

Grumpy attempts to dramatically slam the door as he exits in a huff. But like he can't see reason, he also can't see the little steps blocking the doorway. His failure to rattle the windows and instead jar his ulna (Oh, look at me getting all medical. Cancel calling the midwife; Mrs Grumpy will be around with her forceps disguised as sugar tongs. Less intrusive for one's vagina... Oh dear, I'm off again.) only incites his annoyance more. One-nil to me.

The argument was about a garden trowel, the one Grumpy said I didn't need, and the one I bought that he then uses and hides from me.

Retirement has been like Trowelgate. In the years since Mad Max retired, he's taken things over. The kitchen. The lounge. The main bathroom. My sanity. I bought myself a mini blender, which he uses for his protein smoothies. I bought a blood pressure monitor, which Dr Kildare has commandeered.

That's the tip of the iceberg. Today though, my patience has snapped like the unreliable knicker elastic in eleven-year-old-me's bottle-green gym knickers. Quite simply, the trowel represents the fact that enough is *enough*.

Grumpy has disappeared.

I get back to reading my book.

Half an hour later, he's back...with a new garden trowel that he waves at me like he's a samurai warrior. Warrior, my arse. He's more like a McDonald's waiter. He can't *not* have the last word:

Grumpy & Me

"This is mine! You can keep yours, you miserable old trout."

Oh, Grumpy. No, Grumpy. Trout, is it?

The one thing Grumpy hates is my silent treatment. Well, tickle my fin and call me Fishface. It's like the Arctic in our house right now with the icy atmosphere. He'll need more than a trowel to dig himself out of this one...

They Say Life Begins at Forty

PEOPLE WHO SAY that speak with forked tongues. Grumpy, and men in general, do far better than the fairer sex in the ageing game, although they do end up with ears like African elephants, strangely without the slightest ability to hear. Older men are "distinguished," "rugged," and "charmers," while old ladies "batty," "bags," and, at the very, very best, "cougars." The saying should be " Life begins to fucking fall apart at forty."

I have already drawn your attention to the fact we deflate with age, those with boobies deflating at a faster rate than those growing elephant ears. Except for Mick Jagger. Shit, somebody stuck a few pins in him early in life–he looked like a shrivelled balloon years ago. I have already forewarned you that the hair that grew in hidden gardens sheds its leaves and takes root in random places on your very unlucky face. And then, when you think life has been as cruel as it can to your body, you start to pee yourself.

Last night, Grumpy decided that he needed more blankets on the bed. The blankets are stored in a box on top of the wardrobe. He has had all day to assess the chill and retrieve blankets, but no, he does it when I'm already in bed, on the cusp of snoozing-sleep. He cannot be arsed to get the steps or a chair. So he climbs on the bed to gain access to the blanket box. In doing so, he steps on my ankle. I kick out as I am somewhat in pain from the ankle-crushing clod. He had been aiming to lean across from the bed to the top of the wardrobe, and my kick caught him unaware. I sit up at the point that he's sliding down the wardrobe doors in his underpants, face-first, arms stretched above him, and catching his chin on the doorknob. He ends up face-down, nose squashed flat on the carpet, with his legs draped up the bed and I hear, "Yousth sthtupid sthod." I am now fully awake, the pain in my ankle forgotten, braying like a donkey and simultaneously peeing myself at the crumpled heap on the floor that is Grumpy.

So, at a quarter to midnight, the whole twatting bed has to be changed, including adding the extra blankets that have been sensibly retrieved using steps. The extra blankets? I will be throwing them off around two a.m., when I overheat. Grumpy is disgusted that I've peed the bed. He refuses to swap sides with me, even though he knows I hate dampness. So I end up blow-drying the mattress and spraying it with new freshness Febreze.

This morning, he finds it hilarious to call me "pissy pants."

Keeping Busy

REMEMBER WHEN YOU were young and you'd spend ages in the school holidays playing with a wooden dolly peg? Making a dress for your new doll with Izal toilet paper, drawing a smiley face that made your teeny wooden doll look like the embryonic love child of Worzel Gummidge and Aunty Sally. The twig that you'd fashion into a gun so you could be like the Lone Ranger, a bow so you could be Robin Hood, a fishing rod so you could fish down the drain or simply drag it along the railings?

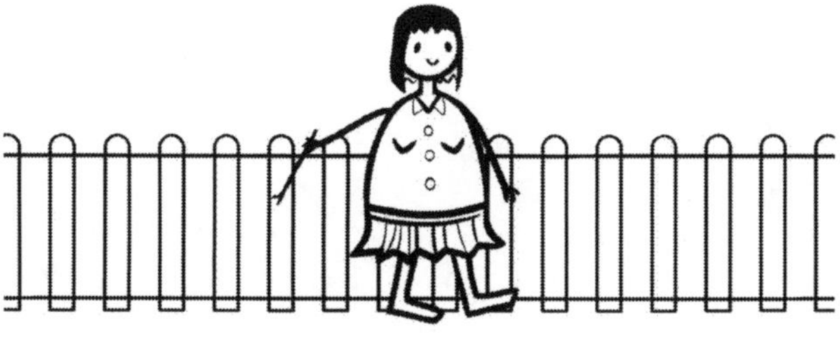

Yep. Shite, but...

If we had that same vivid imagination now and the ability to still accept a twig as a multifunctional, all-purpose action toy, wouldn't crafting, and life in general, be much more fun?

In my never-ending quest to work out the meaning of retirement, I have attempted crafting when I found some old knitting needles. The ones I used to poke my own eyes out when asked if I wanted to do hill-walking. Just like a hill, I don't walk. Nor do I knit. I remember plain. I remember purl. And then I remembered my knitting ability stopped at making a scarf: one nowhere the size of Tom Baker's Dr Who scarf. *That* was a fucking liability, wasn't it? He really should've got that scarf stuck in the Tardis doors at least once before he degenerated. Sorry...regenerated.

I bought a cross-stitch kit. It made me cross. Because I now know I am unable to thread a needle, even one with an eye as big as a cyclops. Twenty minutes I sat there, sucking the end of the thread like a pensioner with a barley twist. All that happened was it got wet. And floppy. Make up your own euphemism about that.

Like most women, I can make something out of nothing. But faced with making a cupcake liner door wreath, I'll admit defeat. Although I did enjoy eating the two-dozen cupcakes...before I realised I was supposed to be gluing unused ones together. When I showed the completed article to Grumpy, he said it looked like the bottom of a bulimic's bin.

I'm still not making any sense out of retirement. The first hurdle was realising I'd been conditioned to conform during the pre-retirement years. Then I slowly grasped I was a creature of habits. I might think I could pack a knapsack and climb Kilimanjaro on a whim, but my whim worried about the laundry. I made lists of interesting places to visit and things I should try, only to discover I wasn't interested enough to try them.

When you read about planning for retirement, it's usually about being financially secure. It doesn't say that it can be lonely, boring, and see you missing work. Nor does it mention your loss of purpose. But like the loss of libido, you will eventually learn to cope. And no, I genuinely don't believe that *many* eighty-year-olds are still sexually active. It takes them a good hour to get their dentures in, so no, I'm not going to visualise them whooping as they undertake #35 of the *Kama Sutra* whilst resting their walking stick against the bedhead (not a euphemism, and I advise you against making up your own in this instance).

So in the meanwhile, until I find my *thing*, I'm going to take a twig and drag it along the local school railings, just because that's something I could be good at.

Staycation Tips for Pensioners

A NICE DAY OUT AT THE BEACH.
Don't be thinking you can still tuck your frock in, or up, the legs of your drawers when going in for a plodge. You'll look like your carer has brought you out for the day to allow your room a good airing. Definitely splurge £5 on a 99 ice cream that used to cost 6d, but lick with a ladylike motion. Any over-relishing as you enjoy the monkey blood could make you look like a Galápagos tortoise. Don't worry about sand in your crevices. It's been a long time since your Nancy Drew had a dermabrasion.

SAFARI PARK.
The one place you can see living things that look as bored as pensioners watching TV adverts. Just like pensioners, the park animals only come alive at feeding time. Just open a packet of chocolate

Hobnobs at bingo to reenact the lions with a side of beef. You will leave the park needing a new car bumper. I'm sure some of the park keepers have trained the monkeys to rip off car parts so that they can sell them on Facebook marketplace. Don't bother with that tea towel memento of a smiling gorilla wearing sunglasses. Just get the photo of your beloved in Skegness printed on one instead. It'll be much cheaper. And way more personal. Don't be tempted to put your hand out of the car window. If the monkeys like windscreen wipers, think how amused they'd be with a spare hand. You only know true love if you need your partner to wipe your bum.

SPEND A DAY MEANDERING THROUGH A FOREST WITH DAPPLED SUNLIGHT DANCING THROUGH THE CANOPY.

Hug a tree. Forage mushrooms. Make a daisy chain. Stand in deer shite. Pierce your big toe with a jagged branch. Get stung by a hornet or twatted by a toy arrow that some eight-year-old would-be Robin Hood is menacing the perceived Prince John's army with. Then explain to the park ranger, a community police officer, and a demonic mother why Little Lord Fauntletwat is now bound tightly to a broad oak. Upside down.

GO ON A STEAM TRAIN WITH AFTERNOON TEA, SO YOU CAN REENACT *THE RAILWAY CHILDREN*.

You always wanted to be Jenny Agutter. But as a child, the nearest you got was looking like you'd rolled *in a* gutter. You'll never forget the thrill of climbing those wooden steps, clinging into the metal rails and standing on a bridge, waiting for the steam trains to pass underneath. Their coal-filled steam filling your lungs and eyes like you'd just finished your tenth Woodbine. Bliss.

SCOTLAND.

A glorious country with majestic lochs and mountains that make you realise how insignificant you are. Tartans that test your eyesight and raggedy Highland cows that graze the land looking proud and handsome. And fucking midges. Marauding little bastards. Given the option of midge bites or rolling naked in thistles, thistles win. What is it that a Scotsman daubs on his Jolly Roger under that kilt to deter the nasty little buggers? But you enjoy the images...and wonder if that's how the Highland Jig came about.

Autumn isn't so far away.

Red Rag

WE HAVE THIS thing going on in our house. When I discover a bed sheet with a hole, my first thought is, "Champion! New dusters." I'll cut the sheet up and store the neat remnants in the cupboard under the sink, which now looks like a storage compartment for Florence of the Nightingale to use on Crimean war casualties. A stash of squares and strips of flannelette. I am *so* happy. I mean, really happy. I love fresh dusters almost as much as I love a fresh pair of absorbent cotton knickers on a summer's day.

Two days later, I go to dust. I open the cupboard to select the correct size material piece for the job. And poof! Not a fucking rag in sight. There are only two of us in this house. Unless there's a ward of sick mice under the floorboards who have just had every one of their two hundred beds changed. I hold an investigation. Grumpy denies everything and anything, including eating four mince pies.

"I know nothing of cloth, for I am not a tailor, and I most definitely did not eat four mince pies with my second cup of Yorkshire Tea this morning, darling wifey."

He may not be a tailor, but he definitely is a tinker, because a thorough search of the garage unearths my spoils. He has hidden the stash in Spider World, just outside my clutches, the conniving C-word.

"Oh, *those*," he bluffs, "I moved them when I tidied under the sink."

After raucously laughing, I challenged him further. "You cleaned under the sink?"

"I did indeed."

"Well, why are there still dirt rings on the shelves?"

"Because I couldn't find a cloth, and you've threatened to sever my testicles if I ever touch your flannels again."

I know he has snaffled my sheeting to use as covers for his recent planting, now that winter has set in. All he had to do was ask. I would have shared. I'm happy to share anything except my food. (Be warned if we ever were marooned on a desert island, and you were my best friend. If I had food, you would not get so much as a sniff of it. I have a figure to maintain. I'd be very sad that you died of starvation, but hey, I'd probably eat you too. Waste not, want not.) However, I know his favourite underpants are freshly laundered: the ones with the hole in the arse. With deft dissecting, I can get four dusters out of them and some buttons for the #justincase button tin I never use. Grumpy was cussing like a sailor as I introduced his Calvins to my secateurs. I spy a win.

Things from the Good Old Days I Thought I'd Never Miss

- ☑ Blocks of mascara you spat into.
- ☑ Bank managers, sat behind their big mahogany desks with eyes like ferrets and daring you to step onto their 100% wool Axminster carpet. Inevitably, bank tellers knew your name and your credit rating. Cash was king. But the bank manager was the emperor. He said "No" long before the computer ever did.
- ☑ Church bells.
- ☑ Bus conductors. If you thought getting one over on the ferret-faced bank manager was difficult, try pulling the wool over the alligator eyes of the conductor on the No.64 bus. Ye gads, they could sniff empty pockets at one hundred yards. You might sneak on the bus while they were fighting through the smoke on the top deck to work every bugger's ticket,

but they'd have you off at the next stop if you couldn't pay the thrupence fare.

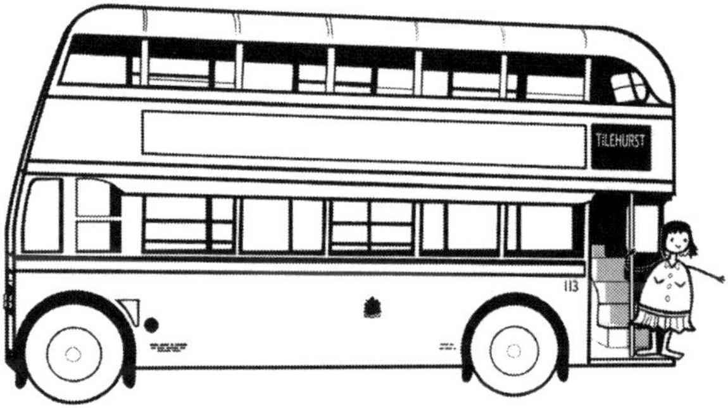

- ☑ The sound of a hand-written letter plopping onto the doormat.
- ☑ Cinema usherettes: cousins of the bus conductor, only with nastier DNA. They ruled the auditorium with only a flashlight and a "Sshh!" as their weapons. Closely related to the librarian. If you spoke out of term during *Gone with the Wind*, you were out sharpish before the interval and the chance to get a tub of ice cream from the lady carrying the tray of refreshments just under her bosoms.
- ☑ Adults being in charge.

Grumpy & Me

- ☑ Everything being sold in brown paper bags. Or wrapped in newspaper. Or carried home in your own jugs or pots.
- ☑ Children being seen and not heard.
- ☑ Twin sets. Sets of Pearls. Brooches. Pinnies. Headscarves. In general, despite not spending a fortune, how much care people seemed to take in their appearance. Sunday best for want of a better phrase. Although the hair curlers under the headscarf, which never appeared to come out except on a Saturday night, was the one exception to the rule.
- ☑ The scent of Sunday roasts filling the street.
- ☑ Taxi drivers who exited their car, knocked on your door, and carried your bags. Getting a modern-day taxi driver to exit his car is like expecting a teenager to voluntarily get out of bed before mid-afternoon.
- ☑ Doctors. I know we still have them. But nowadays, they're rarer than rocking horse shite.
- ☑ Working men's clubs. Not a lot of them about either.
- ☑ My youth...

Male Retirement Phrases Asked and Answered

WHAT ARE WE DOING TODAY?"

Suddenly, you have no real plans. The male is happy to sit all day eating, reading the newspaper, or, if they're trying to get into your good books after being a complete twat, tinkering with a tool somewhere. Usually, the wrong tool at the wrong problem. By asking this question, they're calculating the amount of freedom they have, in which they plan to do nothing. Happily.

You mumble, "I'm not sure what you're doing, Knacker Ned, but I'm researching euthanasia, and one-way EasyJet flights to Switzerland," but decide on a visit to the local National Trust instead.

"WHERE ARE YOU, MY PRECIOUS?"

You're likely to be quietly hiding in the bathroom with your iPad and the door locked. You may be sucking on a Kit Kat, depending on where you are in this month's diet phase. This phrase is usually bred from male hunger pains. They can see there's food in the fridge but are unsure what is grazing foodstuff and what is designated as meal foodstuff. On several occasions in the early days of retirement, they will have eaten half a cooked chicken ready for lunchtime sandwiches and curry dinner as a snack, then wonder why you, on finding them picking the parson's nose out of their teeth, go off like Kim Jong Un. It can also be used when they're looking for their weekly change into clean underpants, and they cannot remember which drawer their drawers are in.

"Shall we have a nice run to the garden centre?"

Oh fuck, this old chestnut. You would rather have a hip replacement without anaesthetic carried out by a qualified charlatan on a wet Monday morning. Old men adore garden centres. It's the only way they can sow their seed in their twilight years. You could feign a heart attack, but I doubt you'll have the energy. I suggest you do a trade-off. One new feather-filled cushion from Tacky Max equals one hour-long garden centre visit without moaning.

Grumpy & Me

"We still have half a cabbage left. What are you going to do with it?"

Just when did my life turn into making something out of nothing? I used to be able to do mental arithmetic, for fuck's sake. I know where I would like to shove the cabbage to slowly broil, but instead I reply, "Shred it, braise it, add flaked almonds and cream, and have it with the cold ham," knowing full well you have neither flaked almonds or fresh cream in the fridge, but hey, by dinner time, he will have forgotten what you had said anyway.

"Shall we have an early night?"

Absolutely not an invitation to reintroduce Roger to Nancy. They've not been on speaking terms since 1983. Nancy's lips remain firmly closed. The reason for this suggestion will be because you have both fallen asleep watching *Gogglebox* until one of you loudly snorted, snored, or farted.

"I love you."

This has to be 100% true, otherwise, within the first three months of retirement, you would have packed your bags and unsuccessfully tried to move in with your married children, accidentally pushed them inside the fridge freezer, and sat on the lid eating a Magnum, then suggested a trip to Alnwick Poison Garden and took some cuttings off the atropa belladonna whilst nobody was watching, or ran off to London in search of Tom *Delish* Hardy.

'Tis Often the Little Things in Life That Give Us the Greatest Pleasure

- The alarm trilling at six thirty a.m., then remembering you're retired.
- Finding the last Kit Kat that had dropped behind the cucumber in the fridge. Champion.
- Wearing new pyjamas in winter. Bliss.

Or in Grumpy's case, finding two "poking" sticks. He savours finding such things with the right thickness, bendability, and size for such tasks as:

- Stirring paint, even if he's not planning on actually painting anything in the next year.
- Waving a pornstar-size length willy willy-nilly.
- Poking insects to confirm they're dead and not just pissed wasps in a drunken stupor waiting to attack you.
- A John Wayne-esque shoot out with imaginary Apaches.
- Prodding holes in walls to check how deep

they are to see if he indeed *does* need to mix sand and cement to fill them, just like the wife said, before mice take up residency for winter.

- ♥ Pretending he's a circus lion tamer with the disinterested cat from across the road.
- ♥ Being André Previn and conducting the orchestra and chorus of kniphofia, echinacea and wallflowers.
- ♥ Whittling like an inbred, banjo-playing Deep South America resident clad in dung-gor-ees, y'all.

However, he really, really, really likes them for cattle-prodding Mrs Grumpy's plump rump, which annoys Mrs Grumpy a lot more than it annoys comatose wasps. After the second thrust, Mrs Grumpy warns Mr Grumpy with a guttural growl that scares off the disinterested cat from across the road.

But Mr Grumpy is giddy with excitement at seeing just how far the stick disappears into the flesh of Mrs Grumpy's bottom when she's bending over getting clothes out of the washing machine, when she's bending over to plug the hoover in, and when she's bending over to retrieve a fallen peg in the garden.

He's so pleased with these two amazing, special

poking sticks and the many, many things they're good for. It doesn't help his case that, as Mrs Grumpy turns around to glare at him one final time, his poking stick suddenly morphs into a sorcerer's wand as Mr Grumpy mutters a magic spell to change Mrs Grumpy into "a thirty-year-old blond with an ample bosom and a penchant for stiletto heels and stockings." (Mrs Grumpy has no idea of what use a nubile young thing would be to Twatman, unless she was to tie his shoelaces. And she isn't that sure many young people can actually tie laces anymore.)

"So you have no idea how Mr Grumpy tripped and landed on two garden twigs that are now wedged up his rectum?" asks the very handsome tree surgeon.

"Sorry, I have no idea." Mrs Grumpy smiles. "I was bending over, looking elsewhere at the time."

Mr Grumpy spent the rest of the week walking like Spotty Dog from the Woodentops...with a splinter in his sphincter.

The Food Cupboard

WITHOUT A DOUBT, like many others, I dearly love my better half. I'd be lost without him. However, there are times I look at him, scratch my head, and think, "I picked that specimen out of all the possible others on offer?"

I clearly missed his yellow sticker.

Since he retired, he has placed himself in the role of Keeper of the Pantry. I held that title for forty-eight years. In which time, I kept neat lines of tins, packets, and jars. Soups and beans were to the right. Fruit and custards on the left. I knew how to maintain order. Everything was in its place. And I rotated the goods.

Today, as Grumpy sat reading his paper, I decided we really needed a stock check. I opened the store cupboard. Ye Gads!! This man doesn't know his mushroom soup from his marmalade. It was carnage. And don't get me started on the best before dates.

I felt like Tony Robinson in *Time Team* unearthing Byzantine relics...from Heinz.

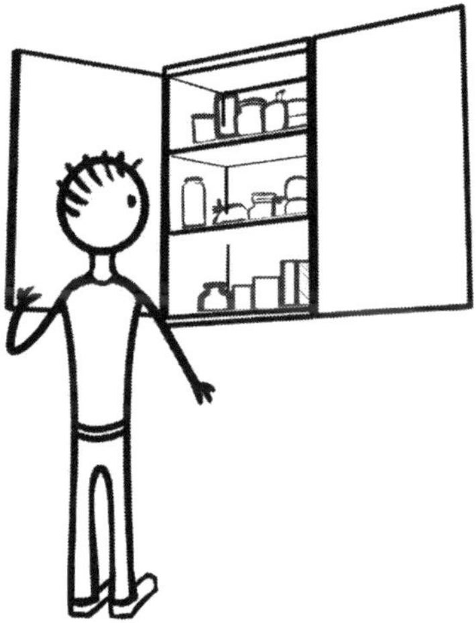

After showing him the goods destined for the bin, he told me, "You're *not* throwing them out. I shall eat them!"

Tonight, he's having Baxter's mulligatawny soup for starter, Portuguese sardines in tomato sauce as a main, with tinned mango and evaporated milk for pudding.

Things People Never Tell You About Getting Old

THE MENOPAUSE BURNED through all your stores of fossil fuel, leaving you susceptible to the cold. Which is why you wear leg warmers. You're not attempting to imitate Irene Cara. The nearest you get to *Flashdance* is if you trip the light fandango when knocking over the bucket while you're washing the floor: "No need to scrub with Flash," as Mrs M used to say.

If you drop food on the floor, it is subject to the three-day rule, because that's how long it'll stay there. Unless you're fortunate enough to own a dog.

At least once a month, you'll leave the house wearing odd shoes. Usually whilst attending a funeral.

You miss both your marbles and pubic hair. Your Nancy Drew now identifies as a bald eagle. Your marbles may have rolled under the sideboard but with your knees, you'll not be checking any time soon.

You carry more drugs than a Mexican mule.

If you're going out for the day, you'll put yourself on a nil-by-mouth restriction. Unless you know where you're going and where the toilets are, including their level of cleanliness. If you're faced with a dirty loo, your bald eagle will adopt hover position, while you hold your frock in your teeth so you can take aim. There's an 80% chance of error in this manoeuvre.

For the first twenty minutes after getting out of bed, you could be mistaken for a Rice Krispy. Congratulations! You are now a blocker of beds, queues, roads, and pavements.

You suddenly start tripping, not because of the drugs (see above), though you'd rather like that. No. It's because, for some reason, fresh air becomes a hazard. If a family member suggests you wear an alarm, kindly tell them to fuck off. It's not you who has an arse the size of a fleet of badly parked BMWs.

You forget things. In which case, they can't have been that important.

You have to part your wrinkles, like Moses did the Red Sea, to apply make-up.

It is impossible not to colour outside the lines of your

lips with No.7's Blush Pink. If you attempt to wear a blusher, you will look like Aunt Sally.

You do *not* like (in no particular order):

☹ A knock on your door
☹ Packaging
☹ The dark
☹ The phone ringing after 5:59 p.m.
☹ Technology
☹ Current "comedy" shows

You *do* like (in no particular order):

☺ Cash
☺ Reruns of *Fawlty Towers* or *Dad's Army*
☺ A nice hand-written letter
☺ A nice box
☺ An electric blanket
☺ Val Doonican

Right, I'm off. *Dad's Army* is on...

Resolutions I Still Haven't Kept

A. Age will be no barrier.

I shall start doing things. Be more adventurous. Erm, except for mountaineering. Or canoeing. Or indeed anything that involves exertion. Being out for more than an hour. Or public transport. Definitely as few people as possible. I think that leaves reading. Yes, I shall read more.

B. Become a club member.

Mm, which club? Golf? Photography? Rambling? Poetry? I shall make new friends. I shall learn new skills. I shall have to make commitments. Adhere to restrictions. Be on time. Nah, I'll join the Tesco Club Card.

C. Be a nicer person.

You know, don't curl your lip at folk who don't have

their purse at hand to pay at the checkout. (Anyone with a purse is over sixty.) Cease the eye-rolling like you're playing eyeball ten-pin bowling when you meet another doddery old bugger blocking the bread aisle. Until you realise you were looking at yourself in a mirror. Don't write "Fuck off" with your tongue on the roof of your mouth when the driver you've just let out from a side road is too weak to raise an arm in acknowledgement.

D. Dickheadinitus is spreading

See C above. Masks will not stop the spread. Social distancing is ineffective. Until a cure is found, I will remember they too are humans. Sub-humans. But nonetheless, I shall be kind. I will not ask if their parents were first cousins.

E. Enjoy life more.

It might mean a move to the Outer Hebrides. Whoa, Trigger. Same clowns, different circus. With thistles. No matter where you attempt to escape, the circus always comes trundling into town.

F. Drink more water.

As impossible as it seems, I do not like water. If Mr God had expected us to drink more water, he'd have given us humps like a camel, not ridiculous ten-gallon Stanley Bottles retailing for £45. Good Lord, when I was a lass, we drank water from a school fountain contaminated by fellow pupils who collectively incubated the bacteria for streptococcus.

G. Exercise more.

It's good for your health. Funny though, chocolate makes me feel way better than twenty squats and wet knickers.

H. Learn something new.

Oh, good, I've done that already! Yesterday, I learned that Gemma the Gob Collins is not the only fat lass that can't stay upright on ice.

I. I will be good.

I will be kind. I will save money. I will lose weight. Next January, I will remember I did none of these things.

J. I shall endeavour to save money.

Mind, the minute I think about saving, I immediately appear to lose pounds without a second thought. If only this happened when I dieted.

K. Sort your life out.

I am not Stacey Solomon...

I'm stopping at K because I realised I hate resolutions.

We Do Nothing to Excess Anymore. Usually...

AWARE THAT, WHILE the head may be willing and the heart eager, the body is a complete twat. There is no other way to describe an ageing body. I don't want to count my blessings that the alternative to an old body is worse; I want Mother Nature to consider her actions and simply stop us decaying after forty-five. Imagine getting to eighty-six and still having bosoms that don't longingly look at the floor like a basset hound searching for a lost treat.

Until such time, you may ignore the body at your peril. It will snap your Achilles tendon, and whilst you're writhing in agony, snap your knicker elastic just for the fun of it.

Even the Pilates teacher is having her big toe pinned with titanium. And she can do the downward dog without breaking either wind or sweat.

In a group of eight OAPs, at least two will have a

body replacement part. Like pin the tail on the donkey, three others will be held together with metal rods. Two will be panicking because they aren't in sight of the loos. And one will be wondering who in buggeration the other seven are.

So, it came to pass we had a lovely family weekend break in the glorious wilds of Northumberland.

Grumpy and me agreed we would have a few drinks and be sensible. Except Grumpy forgets this when he drinks with the big boys. He forgets a bit more by pint three. By an additional half a bottle of white wine and two glasses of red, the fuckwit has amnesia.

He is no longer Grumpy.

He is friends with everyone in the bar. He is Billy Bigballs of the party.

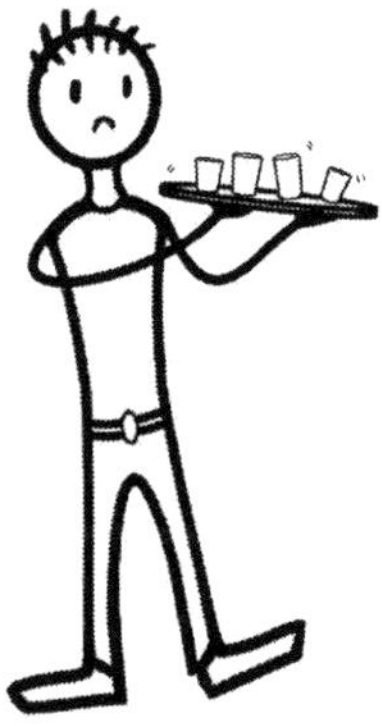

He may have had wine and quaffed ale, but hell, yeah, there's space for more.

When I attempt to quietly caution him about his excess, he's off like Willy Wonka waving a Curly Wurly.

He's sent to the bar to purchase four "baby

Guinness," which he's told should be four "baby Guini" since they're plural. He notices neither staff, family, or other hotel guests stifling laughter. He's rolling like Proud Mary. Eventually he does a French farewell. Or as he calls it "off to the Ponderosa." We do not see him again.

The next morning, Grumpy is back in the room. "Why didn't you stop me?"

I say nothing, which is rare.

Grumpy has dry toast and a hangover for breakfast. We all have a delicious full English.

She who laughed last didn't soak herself in alcohol like the fruit for a Christmas cake.

Your Retirement Based on Your Horoscope

Aries: gifted with child-like enthusiasm

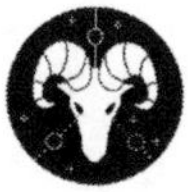

This will ensure that when they end up wearing incontinence pants, they will see the funny side of it.

Taurus: born to find comfort and contentment

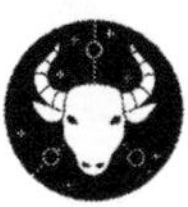

They'll buy one of those electric recliner chairs that do everything except cook your dinner... only to realise it's too expensive to run with the cost of electricity.

Gemini: a student of life

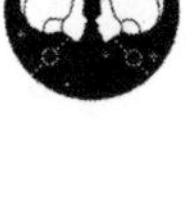

They will have hours to study how to be first out with their dustbin. And why number 46 gets so many deliveries from white vans. And how number 73 can afford to drive an Audi, when they struggle to keep their Toyota Yaris going on £25 worth of petrol a week.

Cancer: born to get in touch with their feelings and channel emotions.

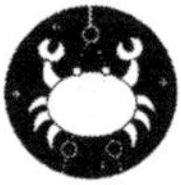

High possibility of spending several hours in a police cell for oversharing with Elsie at the tombola table of the church jumble sale.

Leo: See Me individuals, who need to be recognised as worthy of love, praise, and admiration.

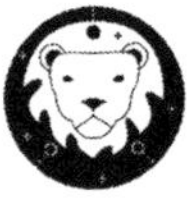

You will rarely spot a grey Leo or one rattling their dentures. They will use Grecian 2000 and Dentafix. And probably Viagra, bought over the counter at Boots, whilst winking at the forty-year-old assistant, who mistakes the wink for a lazy eye and thinks that his only worry should be getting up be from an electric armchair he can't afford the electricity to run.

Virgo: born to embrace the finer details and particulars in life.

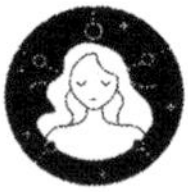

Perfectionists who want everything done right. Will often be found hanging over the garden fence telling the neighbour how to trim their bush. They will always have Hobnobs in their cupboard.

Grumpy & Me

Libra: strive to maintain peace and harmony.

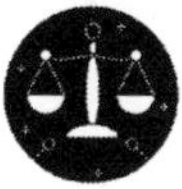

They will join a commune and strip naked. Go vegan and live in Ibiza, with flowers in their thinning hair. And they'll wonder if Scott Mackenzie ever did get to San Francisco. They'd like to teach the world to sing.

Scorpio: driven by passion with an emotional nature.

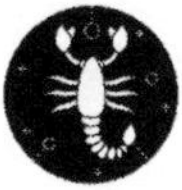

Do not like routines. Sometimes they will put their bins out the night before the collection day just to upset Colin the Gemini at No.42. They may be driven by passion, but they ride in a Ford Fiesta.

Sagittarius: looking for personal and philosophical truths. Restless and in need of freedom.

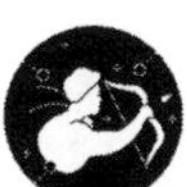

The Judith Chalmers of the OAP world. Can sniff a 5* all-inclusive holiday deal faster than Mr Leo can feel a stirring in his loins, which is simply because his wife swapped their laundry detergent. Will constantly seek freedom, as long as they're home by six p.m.

Capricorn: born to work. Ambitious and resourceful.

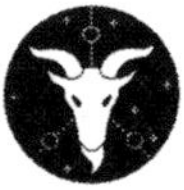

This group will be found wandering in B&Q, Asda, and local garden centres, wearing the company apron, shirt, fleece, and a vacant look when poised with a question. Greta Thunderthighs is also a Capricorn, can you imagine her being kidnapped? Good Lord, the kidnappers would pay a ransom to have this little madam removed tout suite.

Aquarius: born to work for a cause and collaborate with groups of people.

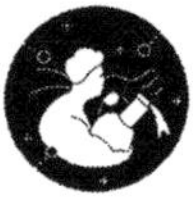

Friendly intellectuals. Will be founding member of the Parish Council, The Ramblers of the North West, Greenpeace, The Farmers Arms Pub Quiz Team, Save our Pole Dancers, Tinder, and can be seen at Mecca Bingo every Tuesday.

Pisces: born to embrace creativity, to reach beyond what is tangible. Dreamers.

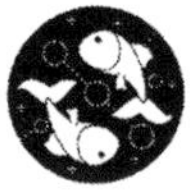

Will spend their pension pot on a revamped Volkswagon caravette they call Sandra. After his mother. They will be on the road for nine months out of the year. But not outside the U.K. They are not kind of dreamers who want to travel anywhere their pension might be frozen, like their arses are in October at Whitby.

Happiness Doesn't Disappear as We Age

IT HIBERNATES. LIKE a fat, jolly rolled-up hedgehog stuffed full of worms.

We grow up knowing who we are. We come to terms with relationships and parenting. We balance books, emotions, and the question "What's for dinner tonight?" Where we used to dance around our teenage bedroom singing to The Four Preps' "Big Man" into a can of Aqua Net, we ended up singing the blues when we suffered empty nesting.

When we should be off spending the Gusset Gremlins' inheritance, we're taking a guilt trip instead. It's a bit like visiting Benidorm. We carry around way too much baggage and allow it to stack up in the hallway of our mind, because we can't be arsed to empty it. So it blocks our imagination, which is why it's bubble and squeak on Monday, fish on Friday and in between, as my mother used to say, "shit, shite, and cacky." Which pretty much summed up my mam's culinary skills.

We still focus way too much on conforming. With age comes great wisdom, little enthusiasm, and less motivation, which fuckity fucked right off when the final crow stamped its feet around your eyes for the last time. Of course, there will always be Brenda and Jimmy who, if they aren't cruising around the Arctic Circle like a pair of beluga whales, are donning cycling shorts and speeding around Ben Nevis with Jimmy's Jolly Roger chaffing in his Lycra, and Brenda having good vibrations from her generously stuffed cycle seat. All they're leaving their offspring is the funeral bill. Few of us have any inclination to follow suit.

We're now at the age when we should absolutely be wasting time on frivolities. I read that the average six-year-olds laugh 200-300 times a day. Maybe that's why, by the age of seventy, the laughs have all but dried up.

When did you last sing out loud? Walk on wet grass in bare feet? Buy yourself some flowers? Chew bubble gum? Draw a picture? Say no if you don't want to do something? After all, no bugger's going to make us sit on the naughty step, because they know full well they'd have to help us get back up and risk putting their back out.

To live like a child, we need to be a little bit childish... Let's rebirth mirth.

A-Z of Surprises of Retirement

A. Any day

Could it be Friday? Tuesday? Wednesday?

B. Biscuits, assorted

Bourbons, Hobnobs, Kit Kats, Wagon Wheels, custard creams. You have to have biscuits with the twenty cups of tea and coffee you consume daily. Hide the good ones behind the cabbage in the fridge, in case the family pop in.

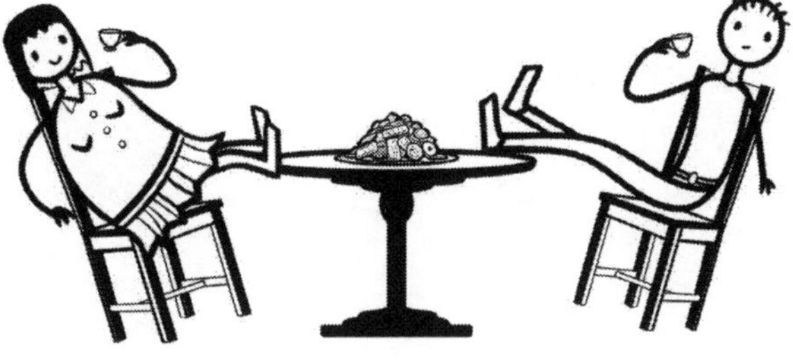

C. Chemist

You need so many medicines to keep you functioning that your airing cupboard is stocked with more drugs than a Mexican Mule. Also known as the John Travolta Cupboard: Staying Alive.

D. Daft

You're not as daft as they think. They're the ones taking you to the doctor/hospital/dentist/chiropodist/ shop on their day off.

E. Eating

Is the new sex.

F. Farting

Sneaky, stinky buggers that pop out at will. Simply look blank. No one will suspect it was you.

G. Garden Centres

Free respite care with flowers.

H. Homes

For the Caring of. Not going in one anytime soon. Hell, no!

I. Interest

Hard to maintain. Often results in Z (below).

J. Joining

The National Trust (no discount, robbing highwaymen bastards). W.I. Bowling. Gym. B&Q discounts. Senior rail travel. Local ramblers. Anything except fucking depressing Weight Watchers.

K. Kilo—the fuck it is

We still shop in British pounds and ounces.

L. Limits: know them

No one has auburn hair and all their own thirty-two teeth at seventy.

M. Money

The only reason a twenty-year-old blond with an IQ is with a sixty-year-old man.

N. Nose

Does more running than Mo Farah and Zola Budd put together.

O. Other people
Really trigger the getting on of your tits.

P. Pension
Fucking Joke.

Q. Quick
A challenge of epic proportions.

R. Remember
Haha haha haha... No.

S. Sex
See R above.

T. Teeth
If they're not in the pot where you put them, where the hell are they?

U. Underwear
The thicker the gusset, the lesser the worry about sneezing.

Grumpy & Me

V. Vajazzle

Finding biscuit crumbs in your knickers stuck to your lady garden when you undress.

W. Wee

Four times an hour between the hours of sunset and sunrise. See B.

X. X-files

Because, at times, you'd swear you were living with an alien.

Y. Your teeth

Ah, there they are! You found them in the butter dish. Lovely pattern on the butter though, eh?

Z. Zzzzz

D. I. Why

I'VE GOT TWO old metal garden chairs that are really comfortable, despite the fact that they leave my bum embossed with a harlequin pattern. I expect that's because my plump rump oozes through the holes like fruit pulp out of a colander.

Every year, I repaint them. It used to take me a couple of hours. Now, each one takes a couple of days.

Grumpy knows when I'm painting them, because I tell him. Further evidence of this is they've moved, and there's paint nearby, as well as a little fat woman who's huffing and puffing like she's reenacting a scene from *The Three Little Pigs*...or a really ham porno movie.

Yesterday, I did the arms of the chairs. I wander off after I've finished to sit in the shade. Well, bugger me (not a request, this isn't *Only Fans*) if a little robin doesn't fly down and clag itself to one of the freshly painted arms. I panic. Quietly. I don't want it to take off and leave its legs behind. I'll end up on *Spring Watch*, with viewers being told about the little robin with prosthetic legs, and all the blame will be on me. I'm just hearing Chris Packham using his stern voice in my direction when the robin simply flies off. It had the whole garden full of trees with branches to use, but no, it opted for a freshly painted chair. It's like that person who has a completely empty waiting room before them and sits down right next to you, the only other person there. They end up three inches from your spare tyre that, up until this point, was just dangling there minding its own business. Now, you dare not breathe for fear that the exhale breath will make your flesh undulate and caress your overly close companion. Body parts are like your last Rolo—not made for sharing. Well, at least not in a waiting room.

I'm finished for the day.

Next day, I continue and paint the back and the seat. I'm talking to Grumpy while I'm painting. In the main, the chat involves me telling him where I'll paint a big black hole if he doesn't stop giving me "tips" on my technique.

Grumpy & Me

He baits me like the grizzly I am.

I do the same as yesterday. Off into the shade to wait for paint to dry, ready to chase any dopey robin with shiny black feet that comes close.

As I take my seat, Grumpy takes his.

On the newly painted chair. Fucking bird brain. "The chair! The chair!" You know what he says?

"Correct! Give Grizzly Adams a coconut. It is indeed a chair!"

He thinks he's funny. What happens to them in their dotage that they think they're Chubby Brown? When instead they're Podgy Grey.

I leave him sat there, waiting to see if any loose change will eventually clatter to the ground.

Five minutes later, the penny drops. He jumps up with the chair stuck to his trousers. Now *that's* funny.

Things You Say When You Don't Know What to Say

"I'll make a nice cup of tea."

Yep, that'll do the trick. Arm hanging off? Builders brew. Severed artery? Earl Grey. Hostage situation? Herbal. There's tea for every eventuality. And if there's a chance of a chocolate biscuit, there's absolutely nothing to worry about.

"We'll be fine."

Relevant if the Boeing 747 you're sat in is taking a nosedive into the Atlantic, or if your car has broken down in the outback and a skinny bloke in tatty dungarees is plucking the chords of "Duelling Banjos" with his marra, while you're trying to assess if his lazy eye is looking at you or eyeing the hog wallowing in the mud.

"I told you so." (feminine)

She did. You can't argue. You could, but you really shouldn't. It'll end in tears. Yours.

"I TOLD YOU SO." (MASCULINE)

He did. But you'll argue black and white until he caves in and forgets he warned you in the first place.

"GREAT!"

Whatever has just happened is absolutely *not* great.

"OH, IS THAT THE TIME?"

This is code for "Quick, time for a sharp exit." Not to be confused with the other party actually needing to clarify what time it is or needing to synchronise watches. Although occasionally, it could mean they've just purchased an Apple Watch and are showing the fuck off.

"MAYBE."

Not a cat in hell's chance.

"IT'S PAST MY BEDTIME."

Whatever you're going to ask, or expect of me, it's a no. My pyjamas are busy warming through to body temperature on the radiator.

"YES!"

No. Never.

Grumpy & Me

"I DIDN'T EXPECT THAT."

Erm, you probably did. You just hoped it wouldn't happen when you were all on the same continent.

"HELLO!"

Fuck right off.

"IS THAT YOURS/ARE YOU WITH THEM?"

Used in reference to whom the individual is with, regardless of whether that be a newborn in a perambulator or adult "companion." Urgh! Make it stop! Someone's been beaten with the ugly stick. My eyes hurt.

"I THINK YOU SHOULD SLEEP ON IT."

They aren't referring to a Slumberdown mattress. They're hoping you'll come to your senses somewhere between right now and 5:32 a.m.

"SHOULDN'T COMPLAIN."

But, oh, they will.

"I DIDN'T NOTICE."

They most definitely did.

"EVERYTHING OKAY?"

This is only ever said when the atmosphere is crackling with tension, and no one is making eye contact with anyone who doesn't happen to be a dog. Even the dog will be attempting to leave the room. Of course, no one will answer, because anything, literally anything, will be used against you at a later date.

Sometimes silence is golden.

There is No Easy Way to Put This

RETIRED OLD MEN are twats.

For years, the house was somewhere they came back to after work, to leave empty toilet rolls in their wake after peeing on the toilet seat, discarding their dirty underpants beside the laundry bin, and asking, "What's to eat?"

Two years into retirement and they morph into Kim Woodburn, with very similar personality traits. I've heard similar stories from others, whose spouses suddenly decide they know better than the lady of the house.

At first, it looks like they're being helpful. You're thrilled. It's been a long time coming. But, like ants, they start by infiltrating your kitchen. Leave them to it and in the next calendar month, they'll be rearranging your knicker drawer.

"The big pan doesn't go there!" he tells me.

"Eh? But it's the 'pan drawer.'"

"Not anymore. This kitchen is a logistical nightmare. I'll sort it!"

Dick Head has nominated himself Butler of the Pantry. Which leaves me as the scullery maid.

"I've rearranged the cushions. Your colour combination was a bit extreme."

Not as extreme as my colourful language. Dick Turpin takes the cushions. Every morning, I put the cushions back. Correctly.

"My" food has been rearranged to the equivalent of the reduced shelf status of the supermarket, but in the kitchen cupboard, King Dick's is in premier position. There is a new head chef in the kitchen. I'm now the Sue chef (or however it is you spell it).

There was an incident in the bedroom that involved a pillow after housekeeping's new self-appointed head honcho said, "Throws should be thrown...in the bin." I don't know what the fuss was about; he's always said he can hold his breath for ages.

My towel languishes in a crumpled heap after being deposed in the bathroom. Dick Tayter's has a double hook...to itself.

I'm like an extra in the remake of *Sleeping with the Enemy*.

Grumpy & Me

Well, today, I've carried out a coup. While Dick Tracy was sleeping, normal service has been resumed. I'm not that bad though. I've allowed him to keep a couple of the changes though–the underpants going in the wash basket for one.

I lapsed and allowed him to take over. An Englishman's home may be his castle. But it takes a queen to run it. No more dicking around.

It's a good job we love them. Apparently.

A Year of Retirement

AUTUMN

Grumpy retired as autumn colours burst on the trees. What plans we had. What japes we would have. Picnic in Tatton Park on tartan rugs, wrapped up warm to keep the chill at bay. Hearty soups. Crusty bread. Freedom. No work. We could lie in bed till noon. We would join the National Trust. Try new hobbies. Have little trips away. Tra la la la la.

We tried lying in bed till midday. We ended up with sore arthritic hips. For some reason, our snoring hit a crescendo. Death threats were muttered under the eiderdown. We became more tired than we ever were working.

We googled National Trust. It came up under "Highwaymen Robbing Bastards." We cancelled the picnics in Tatton Park. We both agreed it would be no fun sitting on a tartan blanket laid over deer shit, whilst munching our egg and cress sandwiches. Grumpy remembered "East, west, home is best" and declared he loved being at home. We discussed this.

WINTER

We would cosy up on cashmere blankets I'd purchased at TK Maxx. We would snooze on feather pillows in the afternoon. We would go out Christmas shopping together while everyone else was at work, and we would chortle at that fact. Being together would be such fun. Warm and cosy. We would hand-craft Christmas decorations.

Grumpy did not like Tacky Max. He didn't like me going to Tacky Max either. He said my eyes glazed over, and I whimpered with pleasure as I stroked the downy soft throws and cushions. He asked why we needed to buy Christmas presents. We were retired now and had no disposable income. And why are the shops full of people who should be at work? By the end of winter, I realised Grumpy's most used word was now "Why?" Closely followed by "No." The getting-on of my tits was starting. More often than I should have, I fantasised about decking Grumpy rather than the halls. I made a rather fetching, shitty twig Christmas tree that Grumpy dismantled and used to stir paint pots. Twat.

SPRING

A fresh start. We would complete all the jobs that needed doing. Grumpy would join a gym. I would join the library and maybe a bowls club. We would detox. We would go fell walking. Out with the old, and in with the new. Grumpy would take me to the garden centre to pick flowers for the new patio.

When Grumpy found out how much it cost to join a gym, he almost had a coronary. He rummaged around and found all his old para uniform (circa 1970), found his first log, and went training alone in the country lanes. I refused to go fell walking after I found a fucking huge spider in my boots (circa 1996). I became allergic to garden centres and the scent of moth balls emanating from the Zimmer generation. When Grumpy would utter those immortal words, "What are we dong today, my precious?" I would say that I wasn't sure what he had planned, but a) he was *not* joining me, b) I was definitely positive I did *not* want him to join me, and c) he should go play with his log before I twatted him with my car keys. My alcohol intake increased by 55%. I started hiding chocolate. And I fell out with the library over a fucking £10 fine.

SUMMER

We would spend the long summer days quaffing fizz on the terrace. We would eat more salads. We would 100% detox. We would go on bus trips. We would start going to the local pub on Friday nights again. Grumpy would go to afternoon cinema showings with me. Two become one.

The local pub burned down. We had to build the terrace and garden, either in the monsoons or in the desert heat. The local bus timetable was revamped, and it passes by twice a *week* nowadays. We did go to the cinema once. I ended up with the poops midway through *Wonder Woman*, and I'm still wondering what happened. I tried salad. It made me hungry. My alcohol consumption increased by a further 20%. I stopped hiding chocolate after a Flake melted in the towel cupboard, reminding me of the cinema trip. I now simply put it in the fridge alongside a picture of a severed penis. We discovered retirement is not for the weak. The only way to cope is to meet up for an hour or so with a G&T around seven p.m.

Grumpy & Me

Things we have discovered this year:

- Groupon.
- Join the National Trust in winter.
- Yellow sticker-surfing.
- Retirement is not for wimps.

Confused Dot Com

GRUMPY CAME BACK early from his run because it was too icy. He said he went a lot further than he intended. Apparently, one slide across the lane sent him off twenty yards in an easterly direction before he was able to grab a bramble bush and bring himself to a standstill. But not before the blackbird he had startled shit down his back.

I told him my mam always said, "Shit for luck," which is one of those sayings I can see absolutely no sense in. Yet still, I say it chirpily to anybody who has just trod in dog shite, fell into a cow pat, got baby poo under their fingernails, or been felled by the Norovirus. Or in this instance, been shit-bombed by a birdie. Shit really does *not* bring you luck.

I also said he was correct to be sensible and curtail his exercise. Because there was no way I was wiping his bum or spoon feeding him if he breaks his wrist in a fall. My love is fickle.

He was still mumbling dark threats as he entered the street, cursing the blackbird for the bramble-speckled shite now solidifying down his backbone, when he stumbled upon the corpse. Strewn across the cobbles lay the body of the workman who had been fashioning a new drive for a neighbour. Dead. As a dodo. Frozen on a patch of half-finished cobbles.

Grumpy is a qualified first aider. He's desperate to shout, "Stand back. Let me through, for I have the gift of medical knowledge and I'm not afraid to use it" in some emergency. He will have you in a splint before anything has been declared broken. He is also a clumsy twat.

We had watched the now apparently dead workman laying the drive for almost six weeks. He was very stout. Stoutness does not allow you to bend. In company, I won't bend over to pick anything less than a fiver up.

This was not a chap best suited to bending over and laying paving stones. His design was all wrong. By day one of week two, he had stopped any pretence of bending and, instead, was lying down to fit each brick. Usually, as you passed by, you knew he was okay, because you could see his chest rise and fall.

Grumpy & Me

Grumpy remarked, "I hope they're not paying him by the fucking hour!" as Bob the Builder lay like a Greek emperor waiting for his grapes to be peeled by a serving wench.

Only today, there was no sign of life when Grumpy saw him. So Grumpy shouted out to him, "Good morning."

No reply.

"Morning!" he shouted louder.

No response.

No movement.

So Grumpy went up behind the body. And kicked it. I would like to say gently, but Grumpy is cack-handed. And footed.

It did the trick.

The man yelped and tugged out his ear plugs.

I was aghast and asked Grumpy, "What did you say to him?"

"I told him the job was coming along nicely, and wasn't it chilly today?"

The Change

ONCE YOU HAVE settled into old age, you're no longer shackled by what others think, nor concerned about "letting yourself go" because you've already gone… around the bend. And up the road. You settle into retirement and accept things will change.

You can no longer hold your spouse's head under the duvet when you have farted. Because you no longer realise when you've let one rip.

You wear matching cardigans…in acrylic, keeping the sparks flying in your marriage.

You cannot remember the name of your two children, but you know every word from the Burl Ives 1960s classic "Ugly Bug Ball."

You both shave on alternate days. Areas of the body undergoing hair removal may vary. Except for the chin area. Always the fucking chin.

If both of you are not sat in your pyjama bottoms by

eight p.m., you're expecting an Amazon delivery.

If both of you are not sat in your pyjamas by ten p.m., your Amazon parcel is around the back in your greenhouse. Or at No.6.

You finish each other's sentences, usually with "fuck off." Expired "Use by" dates satisfy the current level of thrill seeker in you.

You still exchange bodily fluids, just unknowingly. And from different parts of the body than you used to.

You remember so much about decades ago, but you're buggered if you can find your glasses that you had three minutes hence. You'll ask your spouse if they know where your glasses are and, despite your spectacles being on your head and the fact your spouse is looking directly at you, they will be none the wiser. Their look is akin to them being asked how to split the atom. Next Wednesday. If Zumba isn't on.

You have no fear of mouldy bread. It's simply a sign of penicillin. You just cut that bit off and toast it. It won't kill you, and may even clear up that water infection, 'cause you're buggered if you will go to the doctors. How can somebody that looks about eighteen know anything about medicinal issues?

You share an oath that should either one of you die,

the other one will burn, bury, or shred the deceased's underwear after placing their cadaver into their best M&S ones. Actually, it is usually only the female who will insist this is done. The male won't give a shit, shite, or cacky.

Your idea of fun is seeing if you can keep the heating off till November. If you keep your heating in the off position, you can blow your winter fuel allowance on whisky, gin, and a little charabanc trip to Harrogate to have a cup of tea and slice of cake at Betty's Tearoom.

You have no intention of buying a pre-paid funeral plan. Ever. However tempting that free Parker pen offer may be. Your funerals will be the first thing your children, Thingymajig and Whoeveritis, have done for you in years. And wait till they find you've blown all their inheritance at Gala Bingo. Eyes down, look in for two fat ladies searching for the key to the door.

What Grumpy & Me Think Other Pensioners Do

THE TRAVELLERS

Unfettered by the ties of gainful employment and carefully avoiding additional caring duties, you escape to the sun, the arctic chill, or any other of the four corners of the world. He calls you Judith C, and you call him Alan W. He assumes you mean Wicker, but you don't. And he definitely doesn't mean Chalmers. No sooner have your mahogany-toned feet landed back in the UK than you're booking your next trip. You can Samba. You can snorkel. You can ski. You can make a smorgasbord. You can even have sex on the beach...as long as it's in a glass. They can take away your Winter Fuel Allowance, but they'll never take your freedom. You irritate your friends like sand scrunched up your Judith C.

THE UNPAID CHILDMINDERS

Oh, you two cocked your plans up *big* style.

Retirement coincided with daughter Penelope birthing twins. She is now a mummy of four under-fives who are feral. Daddy works away somewhere in Bogotá for a nice company that has a lot of mules. Penelope works with a charity breeding rabbits for farming in Outer Mongolia. She takes her parenting responsibilities very seriously (unlike Kirsty All-Stroppy, who doesn't know the location, location, location of her teenagers). Penelope doesn't want just anyone looking after her poppets when she's back to work within forty-eight hours of exiting the birthing pool. Now you're so busy smashing organic avocados up that you can't even stay awake to enjoy the over-60s tea dance at the scout hut. You keep up to date with your traveller friends by reading Facebook during the three a.m. feed. And sob.

The Rod Stewarters

You thrive on keeping yourself looking young. Everything, including your arsehole, is bleached a Procol Harum's "Whiter Shade of Pale." You pride yourself on still being in the same size skinny jeans as you wore when you were sixteen. You are sick, but not as in unwell. You drink chilled Budweiser and prosecco, know all the words to Dua Lipa's songs, and can do the dance moves. And you aren't afraid to use them. Not for you an early night, a hot chocolate, and a slather of Deep Heat on your knees. Goodness, no. You're slipping into your leopard-patterned G-string around the same time that your unpaid childminding friends are sterilising the bottles for six-month-old Gillette Mack and his twin Will Kin Sword's eleven p.m. feed. Then you're off, committing murder on the dance floor. Silly old duffers.

THE DIYERS

You two are the home birds. Always feathering your nest. You max out your B&Q Over-60 card to the hilt. Your garage is full of tools (including the man of the house). There is nothing you two cannot extend, paint, drill, or reupholster. You know your dado from your dildo. East, west, home is best. You proudly post Facebook photographs of your new water feature. That wank-spanner travelling OAP may show you a picture of his cruise ship, but you can trump that anytime with your new built-in wardrobes with brushed aluminium handles. You drink tea out of home-thrown pottery mugs and nibble on home-made shortbread.

And then there's us. *The eaters...*

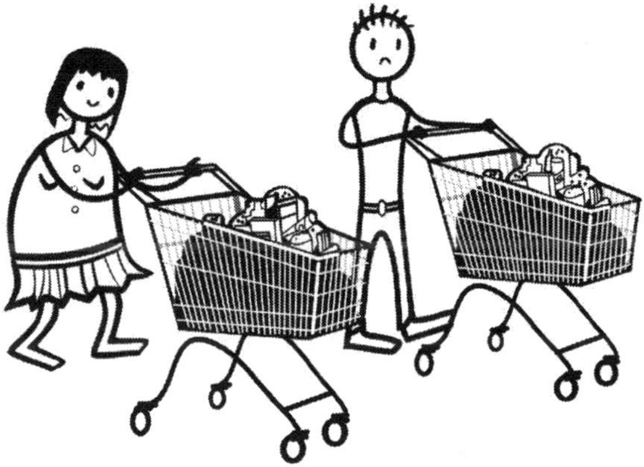

Squabbling

THE FIRST AND last third of your life are pretty much the same. Your main focus is food. Your balance is wobbly. You get frustrated because your vocabulary isn't good enough to make yourself understood. And the middle set of the population think you are either a pain in the arse or "cute."

When we were members of the middle-know-it-all-self-satisfied-twatty-panting age, we thought exactly the same. The thing is you never think you'll get old. You'll never tell the same story more than once or forget the word for umbrella, or have a crumbly hip. That's what you think, smart arse. One day, you will reach the grand old age of #whathefuck. Quite by accident. Yesterday, you were driving to work thinking how much you hate your boss for refusing your holiday request due to "business needs," but today, you've retired, and your boss can kiss your big fat sit-at-home-all-day arse. Champion.

Retirement is a bit like that period a week ago. Remember? Post-Christmas week. You have no idea what day it is and where the fuck all your money went. And you're stuck in the house with a strange relative who seems to constantly be in your fridge or sat on your loo.

Did I also warn you that in both of these ages, you squabble a lot? About anything.

Yesterday, we had Lime Picklegate, where Grumpy insisted I liked Patak's lime pickle. Except to agitate me even more, he called it Patrick's lime pickle, knowing full well that is not its name. I like Sharwood's lime pickle—not Patak's, nor Patrick's, or even fancy pants Geeta's, who Grumpy enjoys the most. On and on he went, winding me up like a reel of cotton.

It was like watching two three-year-olds row about which Teletubby was the best (La La, obviously), where you know it will either result in violence or one of the perpetrators getting sent to bed.

Not to let the subject lie, this morning I slathered lime pickle under Grumpy's marmalade on toast. I used his *favourite*.

The Television Stopped Working

IT'S LIKE THE rest of the UK in the post-Covid years.

We did like most folk: we turned it off. And on again. We unplugged it. And plugged it in again. We are nothing if not highly technically able.

We changed the batteries in the remote. We had a minor hissy fit and accused each other of breaking it. We turned it off and on again, just to be sure we'd done it right the first time. The television is more militant than the unions. I've got knickers older than this five-year-old television. We decided to switch it off and leave it to consider its actions. We did.

And it didn't.

So we made a cup of tea and ate six biscuits each. We questioned each other like a scene from *Line of Duty*. We established that neither of us can remember what we did ten minutes ago. Both of us denied attacking the TV. Grumpy said he knew for sure he hadn't, because he'd not been watching anything political. We reset the remote, the TV, and our frame of mind. We'd managed without a TV before, and Saturday night TV is shite. Grumpy decided to read. The house is eerily quiet. Until I hear a distant kettle whistling. Except it's not a kettle: Grumpy's nose whistles when he's concentrating.

I scamper off to cogitate. That's when it hits me. We may need a new TV, which means learning to use something new. And worse still, being asked questions from a shop assistant who looks about thirteen (so very young that he's not yet grown spots or whiskers) about OED, 4HD, 8HD, UltraHD, LED, QLED, pixels, definition, and UHT (I thought that was milk).

I miss the days when you just switched things on and off. I learn one up to date acronym, and by the time I've digested it, six more are floating around in fucking cyberspace or the meta-universe. I miss the days when all that was stored in a cloud was rain.

My mam simply walked into a shop and asked for a television. Take that in. The ease of it. A nice man in a brown dust coat delivered it, plugged it in, and showed her where the on/off button was. Not a word about Dolby, just pleasantries about the weather.

Grumpy & Me

Okay, the downside of old televisions was that if you missed an episode of *The Fugitive,* you had to be told what happened by a friend. A catch-up then was a five-minute gossip at the butcher's shop about the fancy man of *her at No.76*, who was all fur coat and no knickers.

Remember, you had to *imagine* what colour Perry Mason's eyes were and simply have faith that Fanny Craddock's famous prawn cocktail was pink. You never knew if Robin Hood's Richard Greene was the same shade as the Sherwood green tights he wore. Because everything shown was in fifty shades of grey. Except for that little white dot that shrank down a hole when your mam switched the telly off quickly at the end of broadcasting for the night, before the national anthem played and every bugger had to stand up.

Sorry, I'm off again... Where was I?

Oh, yes, hiding from *Whistle Down the Wind*, while lamenting the passing of a television. So tomorrow, I'm off to Curry's.

When You're Knee-High to a Grasshopper, Time Has No Meaning

EXCEPT WHEN YOUR belly growls hungrily, or the Land of Nod is whispering sweet nothings and the Sandman is enticing you to sleep.

A hop, skip, and a jump, and you're sent off to school in a uniform so big that you'll trip over it playing skippies in the playground. But you'll eventually grow into it. When you're twelve. A school day lasted twelve hours; and summer, six months; and a spelling test, sixtytwelve hours.

Everyone waits.

For there, their, and they're to make sense. For the bus.

For bigger boobs. To be grown-up. To find love.

To retire.

Everything takes so long.

Until suddenly, you understand the meaning of time. And the crafty bugger loads coal on the engine and ramps said time up to warp factor ten. Suddenly, days whizz past. One day, you're nipping and punching for the first day of the month, the next you're reciting "Thirty days hath September"...to attempt to work out when said month expires. You go to bed in 2017 and wake up in 2022.

In the morning, you wake up and think, "Oh another day in the notch of my life belt," but before you get both socks on, it's supper time.

Babies grow like dandelions overnight. Strangely, so do your toenails. Time doesn't travel alone: it gathers your thoughts and steals them...starting with names. Then it progresses to "Where the fuck did I..."

And before you know it, you realise that calendars are used solely to show the date and time specifically for the fuddy-duddies like you. You like the ones with scenes of mountains and lakes.

The tasks you've done on a loop for several decades begin to grate on you. Cleaning your teeth: boring. Making the bed: incredibly boring. Shopping: excruciatingly boring with a fucking cherry on the top.

What used to take you no time at all now swallows up time like a gannet. Just getting a foot in your knicker leg is akin to the time it takes to do a five-mile hike...

Grumpy & Me

Not that you'd ever know, of course, but Alexa can give you the median.

Time flies when you're enjoying yourself. Does it buggery. When you're having a good time, time itself is immaterial. It's when you've had your time that it wants to escape you, and then you suddenly realise that no one has all the time in the world.

Don't waste it.

Let's Face It

For years, you know your face. You could pick yourself out of an identity parade. You're aware of the teeniest spot eruption. You're devastated by the gang of massive illegally parked spots that emerge on your face in the hours of darkness on the morning of a long-awaited night out. You laugh. You cry. You're puzzled. Your face remains untouched.

You fall out of your teens, your twenties zip by, you get married, have babies, and wait for life *to begin* at forty.

The bastard does just as it says on the tin.

You've just blown out the candles on your cake, and before you've handed a slice over to Chardonnay and Guinness, you wander past the hall mirror and do a double take. You have teeny wrinkles gathered around your eyes. Laughter lines. You take another look, and you can see Granny Ivy in your face, only faintly though, as if an artist has drawn your face over an old painting of her. But duty calls. You have birthday presents to unwrap. You make a mental note to laugh less.

The seasons roll on by.

"Are you as old as Mrs Renton?" asks Chardonnay one school morning.

Mrs Renton lives a few doors down. She's in her sixties. Chardonnay talks to her often because she has a dog. And Chardie wants a dog. Right now, you'd like a dog. To kick. You wait until Chardie has turned her back and flip her the V-sign. At work, you check your face. Those lavatory lights are harsh, aren't they? Your laughter lines are now guffawing geothermal stress lines. Your nose has put on weight. But oddly, your top lip has thinned out...and gained a fringe. The shock turns several hairs grey. You suck in air. You try, and fail, to suck in your belly. Fuckety fuck fuck.

At the weekend, you buy moisturiser, tweezers, hair removal cream, a hair dye, and a pot of expensive foundation. By Wimpy. You've boosted your Boots loyalty card by several hundred points.

Your makeover cracks up your husband. It appears you were slightly overzealous with the tweezers, so you have to replace your eyebrows by painting with numbers. It doesn't help when Guinness asks why your neck is a different colour from your face. Stupidly, you casually ask if he can see any lines on your face. He kindly traces three hundred and forty-seven out for you before he gets bored and goes back to watching *Ben 10*.

You buy a dog. You join a gym. The kids leave school. You wave them off to university. You cry. You're an ugly crier. You go to check your face. As you pass the dog in the hallway, he backs away. How odd. But as you turn, you understand. You're face to face with the mirror. You hear a yelp. Either the dog's or your's. Who's that looking at you? Granny Ivy crossed with Jocelyn Wildenstein? Fuckety all the fucks.

You don't wait until the weekend to make an appointment for Botox, lip fillers, and eyebrow microblading. Your husband says you won't enjoy microlight flying.

But Mother Nature hasn't finished with you yet.

You look fabulous. You're skint. You also need new glasses. You look in the mirror to admire your new face.

You clearly failed to rub that anti-ageing, gravity-defying, high-radiance concealing liquid foundation in properly. You rub several places on your face and then rub so hard that you give yourself a friction burn. And the penny drops. Mother Nature has dusted you with liver spots in the shape of Ursa Major's constellation. Fuckety all the fucking fucks with a cherry on the top. You have so many lines and roundish splodges, your face looks like a half-completed game of noughts and crosses.

At least with the Botox, no one can see you scream.

Grumpy is Taking Me Out

I ASK IF we're going anywhere posh. He tells me to dress casually and smart. Dear me. I'm shocked and surprised. Unless it is to visit the local pub or garden centre, Grumpy rarely suggests a night out.

I wash my face, straighten my hair, and get a hidden purchase out from the back of the wardrobe (#thisoldthingIvehaditforyears). I select a nice bubble gum pink lipstick to match my shoes. Tada.

This is like Christmas Eve.

We head to Knutsford. Amazeballs.

We park the car. I ignore the already forming blister from the new bastarding pink shoes. "Piccolinos?" I squeal. I like a nice pizza and a large glass of chilled white wine. Or six.

"No."

"Old Sessions House?" I like champagne with a freshly caught fish dish. The thought of lobster makes me salivate ever so slightly. He did say he would buy me champagne when I got one thousand likes on my blog.

"No."

"Belle Epoque?" I beg shamelessly. Taster menu. OMG. Yummy, really yummy. Lashings of iced vodka.

"No."

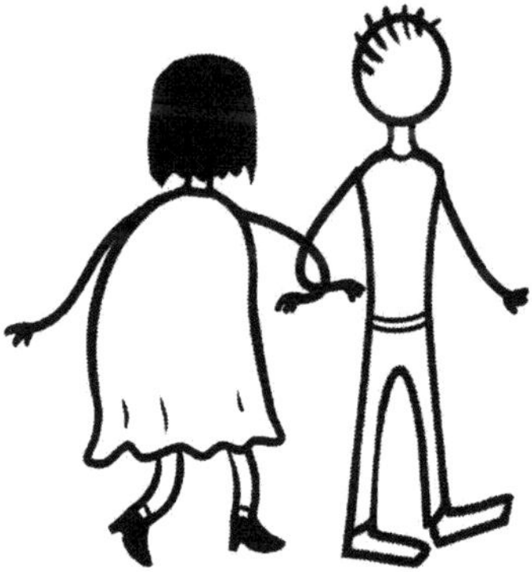

We walked the bottom street and traversed the top street. I'm still ignoring the searing pain from the blister, because I'm getting a treat any time soon. Grumpy is the bestest husband. "The Lost and Found?" Cocktails and carbs. Outside heaters. Hipsters.

Ah, ha. I'd forgotten. The new swankiest restaurant in town has just opened, where just a slither of sea bream costs as much as a Groupon overnight getaway for two. I ignore the fact that I'm now walking like Dick Emery. Grumpy is playing this very cool. This is just like *First Dates*, without that velvet-tongued (and rather fetching) French Maître d', except the restaurant is the surprise. I may have invented a whole new TV show tonight. I could be the new, dulcet-toned Geordie presenter.

Whey aye.

Except we don't head for the new swanky restaurant. Or any other fucking restaurant. Or bastarding bar. Or even the dodgy kebab shop.

Grumpy is taking me to WAITROSE. He's cruising for a bruising, the shit-faced twat. He tells me, with a straight face, he's taking me to do my favourite hobby: yellow sticker-surfing. I'm so paralysed with anger, not to mention pain from the exploding blister, that I say nothing. Not. A. Word.

"But you always say I don't surprise you. You love hunting yellow stickers. We had a nice walk." Yada yada yada.

Mind, on the plus side, I do eventually bag £45 worth of shopping for £14.36. Add to that a saving of more than £80 for the meal I thought I was going to devour. In the end, we've saved over a hundred quid. Plus, the nice chap at the counter was a first aider, and he authorised me a free plaster for the blister the size of a fifty pence on the back of my heel. Champion.

I Used To...

SOMETIMES, WHEN I'M standing with one hand on the bedroom drawers, whilst balancing on one leg, waving like a dandelion clock in the wind, and attempting to get one foot in my knicker leg after thirty-eight failed attempts, I remember that I used to be able to cartwheel.

It doesn't help.

The fact that I *used* to be able to hang upside down on the safety barrier outside the school gates is not lost on me as I struggle to get my right leg into a pair of tights. And fail.

The closest I get to leapfrogging nowadays is when I trip over the remote control that has slid unnoticed onto the floor.

And then it snows.

Suddenly I'm walking like a Geisha girl...one with pelvic floor issues. My mind tells me that small steps will postpone me slipping like a walrus from a rock into the sea.

And it's not even proper snow. Because most of the snowflakes have turned into people. Two inches of snow closed Manchester airport the other day. Two inches. Do they not have shovels? A tub of Saxa salt? A pail of ash? A 1950s school caretaker?

I can remember standing in a crowd of kids from our street, rubbing icy patches on the paths with the soles of our wellies to extend them into a slalom run, knowing as you slid down them later, that if you fell in the right direction, you'd land safely in the privet hedge. If you fell in the other direction, well, you'd bounce back up after a sharp intake of breath and forward roll. Of course, Kitty Holland would usually come out in her slippers and spoil our fun, chasing us, and scattering ashes on our ice rink.

Manchester Airport needs a Kitty Holland.

If the snow was deep, the boys would unscrew the wheels from the boogies, and we'd head for the street near the shops where there was a steep incline with our modified snowmobile dragged along with ragged bits of washing line. To thermal line the wooden plank base, a few of us would bring old annuals. I've sat on a few famous faces in my time.

We knew it was home time when your knickers were wet through and your fingers would no longer freely uncurl...and at least three of your crew had bumps the size of ostrich eggs on their foreheads from hitting lampposts head-on. A cry would go up: "Is the sledge all right?" because while we could cartwheel through the air and slide upside down feeling no pain, the boogie was no way as robust.

By the time you got home, your hands and feet would be burning, while your ears would be ringing from a tongue-lashing for traipsing snow into the kitchen. Your mam would tip the snow out of your wellies and ask you how you got so much in them in the first place. You'd shrug, because you had no idea. You'd been having way too much fun to realise.

Old age is simply payback for living dangerously when we knew no better.

Things That Annoy You as You Age

Packaging

I can guarantee that if you stumbled across the Holy Grail, it wouldn't be packaged as securely as a cellophane-wrapped box of Yorkshire Tea. Whilst many tightly wrapped goods are made to thwart children getting into things that could harm them, they twat the elderly by making any attempt to break the seal lethal. We don't have the teeth, eyesight, or stamina to battle 96% of shrink-wrapped products. It's why most of us are still using implements from the 1960s. The worst we did was key-openers on tins of corned beef. Yes, many of us only have three fingerprints on our leading hand because of that, but we didn't need to be told not to digest battery acid either.

Machines

Show me a user-friendly machine that involves payment, and I'll show my arse in Fenwick's window.

BEING TOLD TO "USE OUR APP."

Kindly take your application and apply it like haemorrhoid cream, minding the gap, to where the sun doesn't shine. For my view on app usability, see above Fenwick's window reference.

GIVE £2 A MONTH FOR DENNIS THE DONKEY

What? So let's get this straight. Poor Dennis gives a lifetime of dedication to his work, then when he's old and knackered, he's simply cast aside, dodgy fetlocks and collapsing hips to boot. Oh, wait. It happens to donkeys too! But seriously, what's with all these charity TV adverts aimed at daytime geriatric viewers. Between Dennis and organising your funeral to take the burden off your family, these canny marketers want to get into your bank account like a love rat eyes your drawers. In the twilight of our years, why can't we just sit with a nice cup of tea and a dunking digestive, watching reruns of *Midsomer Murders* in the afternoon?

BEING INSTRUCTED, "YOU CAN DO IT ONLINE."

Look, Dippy Dora, I'm stood here right in front of you. In real time. But you want me to turn around, go home, crank up my iPad, remember my password, fail three times to get it right, get locked out, ring the helpline, and be told to sort it out next time I'm in the branch? No. I could simply be popping in here for a dose of your sparkling wit and repartee but, on the balance of probability, I'd struggle to find a light behind your eyes, let alone a sparkle. So fire up your Apple Mac, flex your fingers, and make jiggly with completing my transaction.

THE WORLD

You don't know this world. Have you ever abseiled? White water canoed? Foraged?

Look, I gave birth without gas and air, a sound bath, soothing playlist, essential oils, or an epidural. The closest I got to a birthing partner was when the woman from bed nine got up to pee, forgot where she was, and climbed in with me. My Nancy was stitched up without so much as a by your leave. And I couldn't cough for a week without her pursing her lips in case I tore a strip off her. So harness yourself up and don't talk to me about dangerous past times. Our generation had teeth pulled out without anaesthetics, and we finished with a quick swill of iodine. We didn't seek thrills; they found us.

NEWSPAPERS
No longer does what it says on the tin. They may not have *Page 3 Girls* anymore, but it's still full of tits back to front.

NEWSREADERS
Bring back Reginald Bosanquet.

SARCASM
Oh, that's us. We may be passed on the pavement, left behind with technology, and limp like Dennis, but we ace with the sarcasm.

Things You Don't Get Told About Getting Old

YOU WILL QUICKLY fall into a routine, which sets like cement. Any deviation from this routine sees you with overnight insomnia, where you stay awake all night lest you miss tomorrow's 4:30 p.m. appointment. It's no good telling yourself to "get a grip" when you're setting the alarm for five a.m., because you've had a text to say the water board is coming at six p.m. the next day to read the meter. You'll be more wired than an electric fence and not sleep one solitary wink. He'll cancel the appointment at 5:59 p.m.

You used to be fearless. Now you are fear*ful*. You can remember fuck all. Except for bin day.

You no longer have the ability to think. Whereas you used to think on the scale of a blockbuster, you now think for less time than a radio jingle. Your train of thought never leaves the station.

You may scrimp and save, but you always buy a

good quilted three-ply toilet roll. You're very much like the BBC: you constantly repeat yourself.

You have favourites. Chairs. Cups. Biscuits. Children. Hairstyles. Jogging Bottoms. People. Anyone or anything not on your favourite list are collateral damage.

You separate your washing. Not for you, that haphazard toss it all in there together. You have standards. You may no longer use a poss stick and have succumbed to an automatic machine with more buttons than a Pearly Queen, but you still stand in judgement of those lazy trollops whose whites aren't snow white.

You genuinely don't know what you want for Christmas. You might say Tom *Delish* Hardy, but you can't remember for what purpose anymore. Unless he's a good plumber; you always need a good plumber.

You prefer your eggs, bosoms, and scrotum to be free range.

You hide things. To save them or keep them "good," which is why, when you die, piles of £20 notes are hidden in your knicker drawer, you have eight shortbread roundies in tins from 1990 in the cupboard under the stairs, and an array of tablets that cover the

A to Z of illnesses, including a pack for syphilis that you got when you had a nasty bout of sinus trouble. You knew that receptionist never liked you *or* your accent.

If it involves not having an elasticated waistband or a toilet close by, you definitely aren't going.

Your social outings are constrained to medical appointments, church lunches, and supermarket cafes. That way, you can always be home before dark with the curtains shut and the door bolted by seven p.m. sharp.

You will have at least one "for best" outfit, a funeral outfit, something from three decades ago, and several new items with tags on in your wardrobe.

You will have a "reserve" pair of slippers.

You fret about tipping or not tipping the bin men, even though they aren't proper bin men anymore since they wheel the bins and no longer haul them onto their shoulders. This loses them points. Plus, on May 24th, they didn't even empty your bin because you'd accidentally left a black rubbish bag in the wrong bin. Bugger it. No 50p for them this year.

If rolling your eyes was a sport, you'd be an Olympian.

You don't mind folk wearing their heart on their sleeve, but you'd rather they kept their Nancy Drew, Long John Baldry, or Nancy Baldry undercover. In your day, your mam had a saying that cleared a lot of things up for you. "If your aunt had balls, she'd be your uncle." Sorted.

Doing the Messages

GRUMPY NEEDED TO get some timber. I needed to pay some bills.

The arrangement we made was that he would drop me off and pick me up after he'd done his errands.

He took his bank card. He took his glasses. He took his phone. He'd even charged the phone. *And* switched it on. I showed him the road where he could park much cheaper than other places where the local Highwaymen Robbing Bastard Council had tripled the cost of parking. He had coins for the meter. I just love it when a plan comes together.

Grumpy would call me when he'd completed his tasks and was ready and waiting in a parking bay.

I scurried to the bank as fast as my little podgy legs were able...with a detour to M&S for a quick yellow sticker-surf. I'd just fought off the opposition for a reduced chicken and leek pie with butter puff pastry when the call came through. I was "go" for a lift home. Champion. I snaffled a couple more yellow stickers, threw a look of disdain at my nemesis, who was still eyeing my pie, paid, and headed for the spot where Grumpy was waiting.

Shitting hell, I really am out of condition. The slight gradient saw me panting like a cart horse en route to the glue factory. I may have taken a little while longer than a sprightly pensioner of the same age. Fuck.

I see the car. I see it is full of timber. I do not see Grumpy. I assume he's gone off to look for me, so I wait a while by the car. Now this shows how stupid I'm getting. It is a sunny day. The car is parked *exactly* opposite a pub. An old man's pub. Ten minutes pass. Fifteen minutes pass. No Grumpy. I called his phone. No answer. I'm slightly irate. I wait. I ring him. Five more times. I am now steaming like a suet fucking dumpling.

On the sixth call he answers. He simultaneously waves at me from the pub doorway across the road. He's smiling, which means he either has wind, has found a £20 note, or he is twatted.

I go across the road and follow him into the bar. He's on to his third pint and full of the joys of spring. *I'm* dehydrated from all the steaming, and I am full of the

Grumpy & Me

Wrath of the Gods.

It turns out he couldn't hear his phone ringing. Neither could any of the other old men, slurping ale and sucking on pork crackling in the snug. It was only on the sixth call, when the young lady behind the bar shouted loudly at them all, "Whoever has a phone with them needs to check it. A phone is ringing!" Cue five old codgers rummaging around looking for their Nokia 5110, circa 1998.

They all waved at me as I trailed behind Grumpy.

"Bloody phones," one declares. "Impossible to hear."

"What?" said another.

"Eehh?" chirped a third.

"You talking to me?" asked one, appearing to be switching on his hearing aid.

Fucking Hell. Grumpy is downing his beer, clearly afraid I will snatch it from him before he's drained his glass.

I have just walked into a Den of Grumpies. It's scary. I need gin. Lots and lots of gin.

I Ain't Bothered

I CAN'T FOR the life of me remember my mam being bothered about anything as she aged. My dad, on the other hand, found plenty to complain about. I take after him...

I used to get behind the wheel of a car and drive. Now, just getting into the car is like watching Gemma Collins bareback riding a horse. Ugly. I'll have gone a good ten miles before I realise that I've not switched gears, and I can't remember getting to where I am...which I'm not sure is where I want to be. The car behind me worries me if it's too close or too far away. And when I watch some of the orchestral manoeuvres in the dark from other drivers, I wonder if they were taught by Billy Smart. As clowns. I do not like driving.

I used to be able to decide. Now I'm not so sure.

I can remember the days I'd leave the house and not have to return to check that I'd closed the windows, turned the taps off, switched off the cooker, and was wearing knickers. In my defence, lack of a thigh gap does prevent draughts and dribbles, so it's not always immediately obvious.

Occasionally, I don't have the confidence, energy, or time for life.

I regularly choose *not* to do something. Usually, it's because the over-complication of the task is daunting. Like buying train tickets from a machine.

When I say words fail me, I'm not kidding. I can see what I mean, but can I buggery remember the word for it.

I'd love to sit cross-legged on the floor and listen to a story. But it's highly unlikely 911 would ever be able to dislocate my hips and reset me.

I still think I can dance to Shakira...but my hips don't lie.

I can no longer send a greeting card without adding a short story, several abstract doodles, and a polite message for the postman: "Please do not bend." Like he gives a fuck.

I have a terrible urge to shout at the television when the news is on.

I think I'm the only individual who, when being told something weird is called progressive, feels like it's very similar to testing cosmetics on animals. Wrong.

When you can, you don't. You only realise this too late.

The first thing I utter when I check the price of things is "How much?" The second thing is to accuse them of being Highwaymen Robbing Bastards, whose horse Gemma Collins has borrowed to practice bareback riding on.

After all these years, why do I still not know what's for tea?

I miss the days when appliances had less knobs than the House of Lords, when they worked for longer, and were quieter. And didn't shock you nearly half as much.

If someone says, "We must catch up soon," there's a good chance it'll be at a funeral, where, for anyone over forty, you'll assess if their age at death can be calculated as "a good innings."

I look at politicians and think, "Well, now we know what happens when you spare the rod." When they tag a program *reality TV*, it makes me realise they don't live in the real world. I look at our new king, and I'm reminded of George Lazenby in the role of 007.

Thank goodness for chocolate digestives.

Things Pensioners Should Never Say

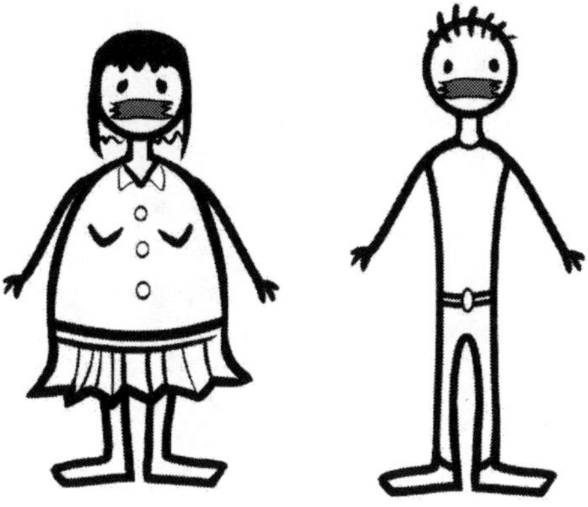

1. "IN MY DAY..."

Oh, Gladys! No, Gladys! You may as well confess to being a Satan worshipper who eats puppies under the light of the silvery moon. Your day has been and gone. You're now excess to requirements. If you continue, you will leave the listener looking like a vacant penny arcade machine, where the jackpot was dropped last Tuesday. Young mothers do not need your words of wisdom in the rearing of children. That's why they have wine. Although you do come in handy for babysitting.

2. "Speak up! What language are you speaking?"

Apparently, it's English, innit? Not as you know it but familiar to a pigeon.

3. "You can call from my land line."

Oh, Maureen. Faced with a telephone with a dial, they'll look at it in the same manner you look at a QR code: *I'm fucked*.

4. "I am seventy-five, you know. I only have one kidney, one and a half lungs, a pacemaker, and diabetes."

Do not even go there. At your age, you're already crumbling faster than the White Cliffs of Dover. The only time this is even slightly useful information is if you have volunteered for medical trials. Or within a group of peers, when you can throw the gauntlet down for a quick game of "Double or Quits" of missing or reduced body parts while waiting for the Mecca Bingo to start. And you'll lose to Bill who is managing with a spleen and one kidney. They don't make them like Bill anymore.

5. "I MIGHT HAVE TOLD YOU THIS ALREADY."

You have. Three times yesterday, once on Wednesday, and again on Friday. And by text on Saturday.

6. "DO YOU NOT HAVE ANY PROPER BREAD?"

Mother's Pride was swallowed whole by Hovis. Modern bread is designed for strong-of-jaw individuals—like sharks. If you want a soft-boiled eggs with soldiers nowadays, you'll be served the equivalent of the SAS: tough, hard, and likely to crack your teeth. It's not called sourdough for nothing. And forget seeded; it is to dentures what sand is to knickers.

7. "THERE IS NO SUCH THING AS A PINEAPPLE OR INDEED MONEY TREE."

Shocked silence.

8. "There you go. Fixed it. Bob's your uncle."
But is he though?

9. "What are you wearing?"
Someone in trainers isn't guaranteed to be about to jog on. Doc Martin will not be making a house call. Vans are not solely used for Amazon deliveries. Budgie smugglers may have nothing to declare or make your eyes water with the contents. Going commando doesn't mean you are enlisting any time soon. Cotton Traders don't. Ted Baker isn't. Superdry gets wet. Barbour doesn't cut hair. Berghaus isn't a home. And Lulu Guinness is not a small Scottish singer shouting to ask if you want a beer.

Funny old world...

How Are You, Hun?

I'M CURRENTLY WALKING around like Matt Dillon's sidekick Chester from *Gunsmoke*. My hips are definitely not lying, as Shakira sang. Instead, they're protesting loudly at my attempts to walk. I look like a galleon that's been hit side on with a barrage of cannonballs and is currently taking in water.

Needless to say, I am a tad grizzly.

In such situations, your better half is always the one most likely to be twatted with an anchor.

"Whatyadoing?" Grumpy asked me as I stood in front of the full-length mirror.

"I'm rubbing Aldi's £1.99 face cream on my face and waiting for my wrinkles to miraculously disappear."

I'll admit that I'm expecting a hell of a lot for something that gives me change from a two-pound coin.

"Take your bra off, and gravity will pull the wrinkles

off your face," the wise one offers.

"Oh, Sir Twattypants, do you think so?" I don't wait for his answer. But I'm certain that all I'll gain from going bra-less is an even bigger waistline on a good day and carbuncles of the knees on others.

Having dealt his beauty advice of the day, Mr Lancôme disappears to get ready for his five-mile run. Sadly, it is not off a three-mile pier into shark-infested waters.

It's a funny one, isn't it, this ageing malarkey? Old men can sprout hair from any body part that isn't their head, they can carry off wrinkles unabashed, and they're at one with the ageing process in general.

You rarely get asked if *their* bum looks big. The buggering menopause doesn't open the tide gate to a flood of aches, pains, and brittle bones for our male counterparts.

I'm now trying my new dress on; it's the new milkmaid style. My milkshakes may not bring all the boys to the yard, but a farmer could well bring a herd of eighty cows and a pail, and I'm set to start a-milking. Grumpy looks at me without seeing. These days, I hover in his blind spot.

"Corset," Grumpy offers as I bend over and wince.

Grumpy & Me

"You need to get one of those whale bone corsets to support your back and hips"

Apparently, I married not only a top cosmetic surgeon, but one who moonlights as a chiropractor, Mr Playtex-Lancôme.

I'm sure that the last time I looked, you couldn't just go online and get a whalebone corset in M&S. Indeed, just attempt to get a firm control bra and computer says, "No." It's also strange that a rather fat creature should have its bones used to make women appear thinner, or less "big-boned." There has to be some irony in there somewhere. Thank goodness those gentle creatures are less at risk from our vanity now.

Grumpy is no Jesus when it comes to helping the slightly sick. In the meanwhile, he has nipped off out, which has given me time to feed his last sausage roll to the birds. Because I didn't have seven loaves and a few small fish.

A to Z of Old Age: Part One

A is for Alzheimer

If you get to K and have forgotten what you're reading about, you're fucked.

B is for Borrowed Time

You are on it.

C is for Cake

Any time, any place. You don't need teeth to devour cake. It gives you a sugar rush, which means you may just get to the toilet in time, at least once in the day, without pissing ever so slightly in your pants.

D is for Dentures

The full set languishing in a tumbler on the bedside cabinet will guarantee that you wake up to a smile every morning.

E is for Eating

Because nature will strip you of any other kind of enjoyment and leave you with this single solitary one. Do not fear. It will enable you to interact with your peers, partners, and shop assistants on heated debates about how to use a full Savoy cabbage inventively in one week, without waste.

F is for Farting

Your bottom suddenly has a mind of its own. You may not talk out of it anymore, like the millennials, but rest assured, your arse will make itself heard. In public, without warning. Never bend over in company, your descent will be declared like the opening of *Space Odyssey*.

G is for Garden Centres

Where you used to love the pub, club, or even the disco, you now let it all hang out around the rhododendron bush, lawn fertiliser (since this is your one remaining chance to propagate any living thing), and summer bedding (on special: buy three for £9).

H is for Happiness

See A above: forget it.

I is for IQ

You used to have one. Now, every word you're looking to use is carefully hidden in your brain for safekeeping. You will only find this word midway through *Midsomer Murders* (the one with John Nettles, the modern one is just not cricket) when, for no reason, it pops into your head, and you have to share it. Then you both miss whodunnit.

J is for "Just a minute."

Which it takes twenty of to complete any task. From getting your arm in a sleeve, to a foot in your knickers. And multiply by three if you're planning to actually go out for the day (shoes, coats, keys, pee, money, glasses, pee, hearing aid, check windows closed, gas off, pee. Fucking KEYS!!)

K is for Karma

When you watch your adult children making a shit job of parenting, DIY, car maintenance, and the laundry. And chuckle.

L is for Loud

You'll be addressed in a loud voice, because it's expected that you have hearing loss. You may do. However, as you've heard it all before, you habitually switch off when younger folk talk to you anyway. Good Lord, they do like the sound of their own voice.

M is for Monday

The only day of the week you can recall. Every other day of the week is simply Groundhog Day.

N is for Ninety

Be careful what you wish for. If you live to ninety, all of your friends will be dead. On the plus side, that means a shorter Christmas card list. But on the minus side, nobody else will know what you're talking about when you mention Laurel & Hardy, writing letters, or telephones with wires.

O is for Old

People will refer to you as old, elderly, stately, wise, or a font of all knowledge. You'll refer to them simply as useless twats. And tell them to "Bugger off." They will laugh at your eccentricities. *You* will laugh when you pee on their toilet seat.

P is for Pyjamas

Flannelette ones with a thick gusset and on by six p.m. prompt.

Q is for Quiet

Nothing about you is quiet anymore. Your nose noisily proclaims you're still breathing (which, in itself, is a relief). Your bones sound like cracking eggshells when you move. You slurp, chomp, chew, and snore like a warthog. There is no such thing as a whisper in any conversation, or an aside, after the age of sixty-five.

R is for Regular

Bowel movements. And in-depth discussions regarding said movements.

S is for Spouse

The one reason you stay alive...so you can see that bastard buried.

T is for Tablets

Hundreds of little pills, capsules, powders, and lotions. You and your spouse have enough drugs to start your own cartel and outsell the Mexican bandits.

U is for Urinary tract

The only pissing about you will now get up to.

V is for Vest

You'll suddenly get a strange desire to start wearing a vest. The male can tuck it around their willy for more absorbency. The female can tuck it under their tits to stop them dropping out underneath their buttoned-up cardigan.

W is for What?

You are constantly bemused, asking what this, that, and the other are. By the time it's fully explained to you (with a quick sketch to shore up the verbal detail), it will take all of five seconds for you to forget.

X is for X-rays

These will increase as you trip over anything and everything from the size of a dog hair. But you do get a nice day out. And tea and biscuits.

Y is for Youth of today

Twats.

Z for Zimmer Frame

You swore you wouldn't be seen dead with one. Yet, here you are, pushing one with a seat, storage, four-wheel drive, and a warning bell. Good Lord, you'll be organising a funeral plan before you know it.

When the Clocks Go Back

WITH THE NIGHTS drawing in, I'm in nesting mode. Grumpy said I was resembling a bald eagle as I clucked around, preparing my side of the sofa to settle my rotund rump upon as lockdown time of 6:01 p.m. approached. My feathers remain unruffled by his observations. We all know what happened to the dodo he's identifying as. My thick fleecy PJs are currently lounging on the bed, expanding after being squished into a teeny drawer for almost six months.

But...

Can I buggery remember where I've stashed the winter cushions, throws, and all things orange. It should be easy. We live in a bungalow.

Clearly, I share my DNA with a squirrel. I bury things. Then I can't recall where they are. Grumpy needs to be on his toes.

I've been looking all day. I decided to have another

check. My mind won't switch off. Usually, I can't get the bugger fired up.

I'm getting annoyed.

Grumpy is like McDonald's. He's *loving it*. He can see no sense in "paraphernalia and trinkets."

Two hours later, in my temper I've managed to pull the place to bits, and I'm trickled with sweat like icing on Chelsea buns. When I decide to lean over to check out the bottom of the wardrobe, my bosoms fling themselves to freedom using the sweat slalom my escaping bodily fluids have created in my décolletage, walloping my jowls with the ferocity of a Will Smith slap. Two can play at that game. I respond in kind. Like Tarzan. A tussle follows as my nipples show themselves for the first time in years and snag inside the broderie anglaise trim of my brassiere. Ye Gads.

I emerge victorious. Nobody makes a tit out of me, although I haven't bedded them back in properly. I'm letting them consider their actions first.

Still inside the wardrobe, I find a new pair of summer sandals I'd forgotten about and four wire coat hangers. It's the hiding place of a collection of the one missing sock from a pair that never makes it back after a hot wash. Oh, and there are our last wills and testaments, all caked in dust. It's like a treasure hunt with shite prizes.

With age comes great confusion. We battle this with routine. Objects go in the same place. There's an aptly named key rack. Lists. Completion of crossword puzzles to keep the brain ticking. Familiarity.

The dislike of change. The love of the deeply embedded habits that we perform without the need for thought. Still...

Grumpy enters the room. "What exactly are you looking for, my little toffee apple?" asks Grumpy. "Erm...are they your nipples?" He recoils.

I give him *the look*.

"Are they in that box atop the wardrobe in the spare room?"

There's a part of me that knows full well he knew that all along. We're ready for you, winter. And the nipples are back in hibernation.

Let's Do a Reverse Cowgirl

SORRY, WRONG BOOK. A reverse A to Z of old age (or something for the weekend)...

Arithmetic. We know how many beans make five and don't need a calculator to sum it up. We know that a gross plus a baker's dozen would give us one-hundred and fifty-seven, and that a furlong isn't a German shepherd dog's coat. We fathomed that out without hiding our light under a bushel.

Bugger off Helen Mirren and all those other "fabulous" old female actresses who make us feel inadequate in our elasticated waisted trousers and Sketcher shoes. Without a make-up artist and good lighting, we could pass you in B&M and not blink. As my mother used to say, "If it wasn't for the weight of her arse, she'd fly."

Cunter, Sursés, Switzerland. You know a good few inhabitants hailing from that part of the world.

Determination. We have it in bucket loads, but we usually have to empty the buckets of the shite we take from some quarters to make room for it.

Eyesight. With ageing, your eyesight does diminish. Although your ability to see through people increases dramatically.

Forgetful. We get out of loads of situations by merely forgetting about them, purposely accidentally mispronouncing words, and using the "daft" card more times than Katie *Tut Tut* Price.

Guilty Pleasure. Nothing gets you going like a nice chocolate biscuit. And a mid-afternoon rerun of *Perry Mason*.

Hots. We still get them. Except the person in question is usually long since dead. Ooh, Paul Newman.

Ice cream. We're now at that age when no fucker

can stop us eating ice cream for breakfast.

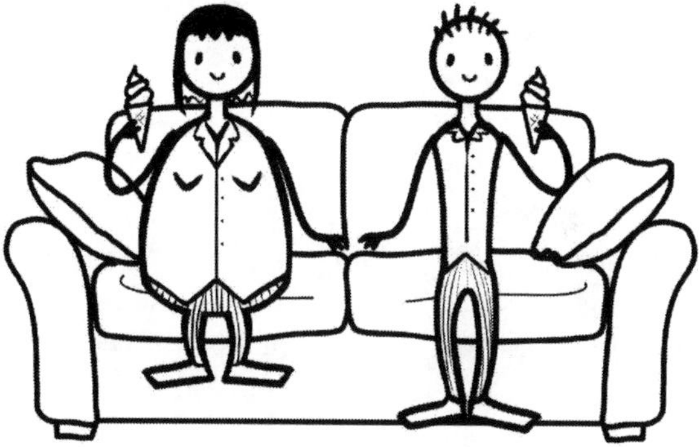

Joints. We know more about joints than any shady street corner drug dealer. Ours creak.

King Charles. No matter how many times you hear his name, you still think, "Who?"

Living. Longer. Eighty is the new sixty, apparently. Years ago, you went into the chemist and came out hiding a packet of condoms. Now, you come out carrying a huge bag of medicines. You're in that chemist so often, they've named a suppository after you. Anything to get you moving along.

Marijuana. Medical reasons thereof. We trip more times when sitting down than being upright with our friendly little stash of pain relief. It's better than an apple a day for keeping the doctor away. And it certainly makes your fairy cakes take flight.

Nancy Drew. While young ladies fear intimate photographs of their ginger snaps sent to boyfriends will find their way onto social media, all Betty has to worry about is if the scan of her Nancy will get sent to the right consultant at the Royal Victoria Hospital.

Octogenarian. When questioned, 30% of men over eighty confirmed they are still virile and actively looking for sex. Unfortunately, they don't know where their wives have put it.

Pops. Just because it pops into your head, it's not okay to let it pop out of your mouth. Who am I kidding? Let it rip, ratchet gob.

Quinoa. Fuck off with your fancy, prancy food stuff and get a bit of Pek chopped pork in a bun.

Realistic. We see folk climbing Kilimanjaro and applaud ourselves for getting a foot into our knickers without holding on to the dressing table.

Shape. You've been trying to get into shape for years. Now you realise you already are: a big round circle shape.

Thermals. Winter survival kit for the elderly. By November, the Febreezing of the gusset isn't working as well as it should. In an attempt to get around this, don't be tempted to spray deodorant close to Nancy Drew; it'll make her eyes smart and lips sting. You'll be walking like John Wayne till Xmas unless you give in and wash them.

U squint at the big light, because it's bright. You squint at people because they're not.

Venting our spleen. Yep, we take no prisoners. We aren't afraid to tackle subjects that other generations won't mention. I mean, come on! What are they going to do? Stick us in prison in a nice warm cell and cook our dinners?

Werther's Originals. Bag of shite.

X-rated films. If they think anyone believes that what that couple are doing is physically possible on an IKEA bed without her having a replacement hip before her 50th birthday, I'll go to the foot of our stairs.

You. Are marvellous. You're mentally stable (mostly), polite, considerate, and you'll occasionally drop a pound in a charity box. So make sure you don't forget to be good to you. In the words of St L'Oreal of The Shampoo: "You're worth it."

Zzzz. We can have a nana nap any time we like.

The Barber

GRUMPY IS OUT.

All is well in my world.

Because there has been drama.

You will by now know Grumpy does not like change. I'd go as far as to say even fresh bedsheets tips his world off kilter. And clean underpants? Well, you can physically see the pain in his arse. Sorry. His face.

So when he went out to his barber (Note: not "men's hairdresser," or "Turkish cosmetologist," or "gent's hairstylist." Barber. As in "of Seville" and Sweeny Todd.) yesterday, he was back quicker than expected.

I will not lie. I like having the house to myself now and again. There is no huffing and puffing that this, that, or the other, is deliberately setting out to ruin his day. I am this and that, the universe and all it entails is the other.

He doesn't have much hair left so he's not away for long.

His hairstyle is now casual "none marauding Viking". Crew cut on the side and back, and what I'd describe as a fluffy feathery look on the top. The feathery top lets him know which way the wind is blowing across his longship. His barber knows exactly how he likes it, 850 AD.

I heard him return.

There was much slamming of doors. His barber has gone to Valhalla.

Well, retirement. In Blackburn. And Grumpy is not happy.

Because not only did he cut his hair he spoke the same language. They put the world to rights as Grumpy sat in the chair. It was something Grumpy looked forward to. And it only cost him £7.

It's funny that, as we age, familiarity no longer breeds contempt. It gives comfort.

When you're young you look forward to "new." Because every new experience is a learning curve. You soak newness up and squish it around your toes. You're not afraid of new. Because if it doesn't work you'll have plenty of time and energy to try something newer. You have a big vacant brain that requires filling. Puberty is the first barrier the young you will hit. When you have to cleanse yourself of childhood and step through the portal of adulthood, where new is introduced to caution and responsibility. The party poopers. Despite the battle, you're still ready for war. You're gathering experiences like Mrs Hinch gathers dust. Woo Hoo.

It's all going so well....

But before you know it, with very many decades of new under your elasticated belt there becomes a point, when, like listening to Donald Trump, you glaze over. And he's neon enough that he should capture your attention.

Your brain capacity is full. It spends a lot of time buffering. And some information held becomes corrupt. So much so it repeats on loop. You've rebooted more times than the average squaddie. Quite frankly, you're outdated. And quietly satisfied with that.

You do not like new. Old is the new new. In fact you can take new and shove it.

The only new you might consider is if they double

dip Hob Nob biscuits on both sides with chocolate. We have reached that point.

I get how Grumpy feels. The thought of a new bra brings me out in hives. He doesn't want a new barber.

But what he wants and needs are two different things. Today he is out looking for a new barber. It will go one of two ways. Fingers crossed Odin is on his side.

A to Z of Old Age: Part Two

A is for Ability

Which, for most things, has fucked right off and left you standing there saying, "Well, I used to be able to..." You can't anymore. And for the love of God, please don't try. A&E waiting times will keep you out long after PJ'o'clock.

B is for Brain

It jumped ship when you were distracted looking for ability.

C is for Cunnilingus

Not the answer to the question, "Name the cheap Irish air carrier know for sly ways of increasing costs," as you insisted at the local pub quiz on Wednesday night. Not only did you lose a vital point and the confidence of three members of the team, but you've also stirred Fred the Quizmaster's unhealthy interest in you.

D is for Downward Dog

You were asked to leave yoga when every attempt at a downward dog made your rectum open and deliver enough gas to knock out a full battalion of fusiliers... not to mention poor seventy-five-year-old Cedric, who stupidly stood next to you in the class.

E is for Ever

Not a lot of it left now.

F is for Future

See E above.

G is for Grey

Hair. Fifty shades thereof, including the thinning pubic ones. Those sprouting in his ears and out of his nose. And those dangling from your chin.

H is for High Heels

You found a pair in the bottom of the wardrobe, only to discover they fit you in the same way Cinderella's shoes fit the Ugly Sisters. They stopped at your bunions, with your little toe hanging over the side like a seasick rodent on a clipper ship. They were as callous to your feelings as the calluses on your sole.

I is for Indigestion

Used to be triggered by food. Now triggered by *News at Ten*.

J is for Jamming

You used to do this with your guitar. Now you stand in front of a row of Hartley's preserves and can't choose between strawberry and raspberry.

K is for Knees

Tricky pair of buggers. When you least expect it, they will lock, leaving you on the floor, up a ladder, sat on the toilet, or in the middle of deadheading...unable to move. Do not antagonise them by making any sudden movements, such as flamenco dancing.

L is for Living

Your battery is currently running at 23%. And dropping.

M is for Money

Tucked under the bed. Behind the clock. In your socks. Fuck the bankers. If they go down, they aren't taking you with them.

N is for Naked

The getting of. A certainty for curing hiccups, although it may trigger heart failure in an unsuspecting window cleaner.

O is for Opening

You can no longer get into packages, especially foodstuffs. You can no longer bite your way into them even if you take your denture out and use them in a sawing motion. You fully believe the theory that the government is behind this attempt to starve old folk to death and reduce the pension drain.

P is for Pants

Big ones. Wide gusset. Strong elastic. Thongs are for choirs. G strings are for the orchestra. French are for those who surrender easily.

Q is for Quick

A challenge of epic proportions.

R is for Running

Apart from your nose, forget it.

S is for Sport

There is no man who looks as stupid as the one participating in a game of walking football.

T is for Tinned Food

You are stocked for Armageddon. Tins, jar, packets, and boxes of stuff, including three jars of kimchi you bought after you saw that lovely Michael Palin eating it. You have absolutely no idea what it is, but it's bound to go with a nice bit of tinned salmon and cucumber one Sunday.

U is for Understanding

You have none left. Nothing makes bastarding sense any more. You're still smarting from being refused a Gingerbread MAN, and instead being offered a "non-standard shade of bread personage of any gender."

V is for Vests

Once the chill of winter sets in, you have these tucked into your knickers, where they remain until spring has been declared.

W is for Wee

You have a cup of tea, you wee. You cough, you wee. You sneeze, you wee. You hurry, you wee. You attempt a star jump, you piss a tsunami down your leggings and into your trainers.

X marks the spot

You have selected your burial plot. High-five yourself for being a landowner at long last.

Y is for Yawn

It must be two of the p.m.

Z is for Zero

The total number of fucks you give at any one time.

It Has Snowed

FROM INSIDE THE house, it's the most wondrous time of the year.

Take a step outside, and anywhere over the age of ten, it is Armageddon.

Grumpy is quite the mountain goat...in both smell and agility. Until he steps on snow. Then suddenly, he morphs into Bambi. He has split his chin and gashed his leg in winters long ago. Now he's older, if he were to slip and break a leg, he would probably die from his injury. Not because it would go gangrenous, but because, trapped in the house with him chuntering on, leg in cast, I would kill him.

Our house is on an incline. This morning, he stepped outside to collect the newspaper, and before my eyes, without uttering a single word, he slid sideways down the drive, past two cars, three shrubs, and one startled sparrow into the middle of the road, doing a superb triple axel in front of the milk float before stopping dead in a frozen tyre track.

"What did you do that for?" I heard myself ask, incredulous. My first thought was to go out and see if he was okay. My second thought was that I was a fucking moron. One: I would ruin my slippers. Two: I would most probably knock him unconscious (despite the fact I know nothing about aerodynamics, I am pretty sure my body mass would be sufficient to travel further and collide with anything obstructing my path. In this instance, Grumpy). And three: I couldn't really be arsed.

So I waved at him.

He waved back. And wobbled.

I did consider shouting, "Do you want to build a snowman?" until he mouthed a silent threat to shove an icicle into some crevice I may or may not have hidden upon my person. He did start off by adding a couple of angry thrusting gesticulations to emphasise the ramming of the icicle in graphic details. But these uncalled-for movements triggered the start of a skid, and his hands involuntarily shot out into open palms to make him look like Marcel Marceau looking for the way out of an igloo in the Land of the Midnight Sun.

This was promising to be quite a show.

By the time I had returned from fetching my cardigan, he was miraculously back in the drive, grasping at the car door handle for dear life and acting as if nothing had happened. Since the neighbour across the road was now outside on perfectly steady feet, Grumpy has managed to remain upright, with his dignity intact and doing his best to look as chilled out as Scott of the Antarctic.

In his absence, I have etched two A4 sheets of paper with a large number three on both. I shall give him his ice dance scores, for technical content and presentation, once he gets back from the shop.

Let it snow, let it snow, let it snow...

Grumpy and Pyjamas

GRUMPY GOT HIS first ever pair of pyjamas at the age of sixty-eight. He has never, ever sat and chilled out or got home after a bad day at work and felt the need to don his PJs and resolve a drama. Or sat and waited for Santa. Or been in hospital (ever) and sniffed his PJs to remind him of the comforting thought of home. Or wore his PJ bottoms back to front when hurriedly answering the door to the postman.

How do you mend a broken heart? PJs.

How do you manage a bad day as a stay-at-home mum with two under-threes? PJs.

How do you manage the guilt of eating three Christmas selection boxes on Halloween? PJs.

In short, he does not understand the medicinal healing power of flannelette night wear.

The purchasing of the PJs was my idea. It got off to a bad start when the shop left the security tags on, and I had to do a twelve-mile return journey. Security tags on PJs: what is the world coming to? But then, if you rely on your PJs as much as the rest of the Western world, I suppose PJs carry the same street value as crack cocaine. Although I wouldn't like to smuggle XL-size PJs up my bum.

It took a while to coax him into his new evening attire. He felt it unnecessary and quite unmanly. For who would run out of the house at midnight and see off would-be burglars or wanton yobs? A man in soft down PJs with a moustache of cocoa around his mouth is clearly not a menacing sight. Then Grumpy realised he could send me outside instead and that would see the fuckers run for their lives, possibly in need of therapy for the foreseeable.

I must confess, I almost bit through my lip when he sashayed into the room with the top tucked into the bottoms and the bottoms, a la Simon Cowell, pulled up to his tonsils. Watching Grumpy trying to look chilled out is disturbing.

"Shitting hell," he declared. "Glasses, hearing aid, gout, a bald patch, and now, fucking pyjamas!"

"At least you still have a walking stick to look forward to. I shall buy you a stout wooden one with a silver deer's head as a handle. You'd like that." I chortle.

He ignored me and slipped one of his slippers off. He loves his slippers the way I love PJs. I hate slippers the way he hates PJs.

He then proceeded to sniff his slipper and proclaimed it to be approaching new slipper season. "These ones smell like ripened Gorgonzola with a hint of farmyard manure."

That's his Christmas present sorted then.

Although I doubt very much he will be participating in the Great Christmas Eve Pyjama Hunt, with willingness, any time soon.

Time

I CAN REMEMBER my ageing dad telling me how many cats had walked past his garden gate, and how many dared to take a step onto the path on any given day. Before he went out and chased them. The intensity of his data collection both amused and baffled me.

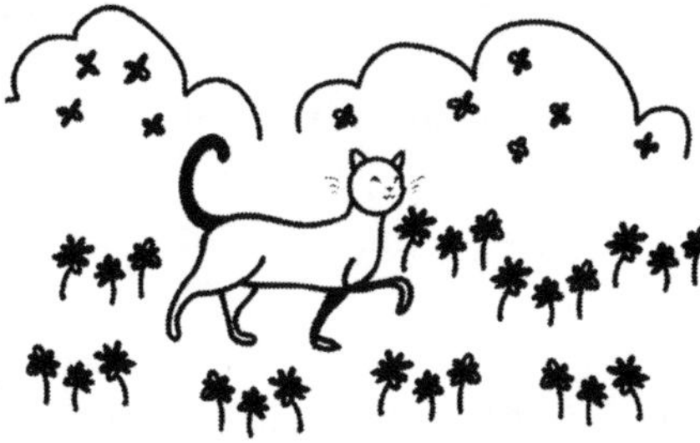

He had too much time on his ex-working man's hands in retirement.

I've told you before that I struggled with retirement. It was like getting the Christmas gift you'd been longing for, only to find you couldn't work out how to use it. Like a pressure cooker. Goodness, they terrified me. Although nowadays, it would be the smart TV. Anyway, you get my drift.

It took a while, but eventually I worked it out. Retirement, not the pressure cooker. After one hiss too many, the pressure cooker went (probably to the Scouts' jumble sale).

Grumpy relaxed into retirement way better than me.

Or so I thought.

This last week, he's been telling me about pigeons, and how they're flying over the garden, landing on the fence, cooing on the rooftops. And reenacting *Love Island*. What pigeons lack in IQ, they make up for in sex drive. A couple of times, I was tempted to go, "Coo!" when he related another fact of the day in the life of a pigeon.

Then I came home to find Grumpy patrolling the tree in our garden armed with a garden cane. A stand-off was taking place. The pigeon would plonk itself on a branch, and Grumpy would wave it on. This went on for most of the afternoon. Watching this, it was difficult to assess who was winning. Then I realised neither party had anything better to do. The pigeon had no pie to be in, and Grumpy had no jobs to do.

I wonder if Sir David the Magnificent Attenborough got his *Planet* series idea from some similar scenario.

Luckily for Grumpy, that's where I come in.

I start cleaning the outside windows. Badly. Nothing works better. Grumpy takes his eye off the pigeon, fidgets a bit, and asks for the cloth. He cleans the windows, to show me how to do them properly. Like I care. I praise him. The pigeon has observed all of this from the safety of his favourite branch in Grumpy's favourite tree.

Then he cooed too loudly, reminding Grumpy how much he hated him, resulting in him launching the sodden chamois cloth in the direction of the coo. That set the cat amongst the pigeons. Paxo the Pigeon (Grumpy is calling him this because he says he needs a good stuffing) took flight. And promptly, with near-perfect aim, shat on the patio doors.

I didn't mean to laugh. But I did. Heartily.

Grumpy spent the rest of the afternoon making a sling shot. Luckily for Paxo, his eyesight isn't as good as it was. And his aim is nowhere as good as the pigeons'.

Isn't retirement grand?

Warning: the Following May Upset Readers of a Delicate Disposition

FOR WHICH, I'M probably sorry. A bit. Nah, just kidding. Don't read the bits that upset you.

What I'd like to know is, if Mr God made us in his own image, and he's been around for ages being all omnipotent (whilst unageing), why did he think us ageing was a good idea?

Got that wrong, Mr God.

I mean, look at Barbie and Ken. They've been around for years and not a wrinkle or worn-out body part between them. Her tits are as pert as ever. Although why it's fine for her to have bosoms, yet her Nancy Drew and his Jolly Roger are literally glossed over has always been an enigma to me.

And let's talk about suffering. You sprinkled us with free will. Champion. Although 75% of us struggle to select from a restaurant menu for fear someone else's choice will be better than our own, while the other 25% let their wife pick for them. Then you think suffering will do us good. From experience, I'd say it's not for me, thank you kindly. Could you possibly pop back to the drawing board and do Version 2.0 of us mortals?

Oh, dear. That went well off the subject, didn't it? It's clear to see that when I do pop my clogs, I'll be spending some time on the naughty step at the Pearly Gates before I gain access.

Now, where was I?

Ah, yes. We've been decorating the kitchen.

After a fraught week, I think I should pass on what I have learned from this experience in an *A to Z of Decorating with Your OAP Husband*:

A) Don't fucking do it

B) Just don't fucking do it

C) A swear word you dislike intensely yet have said it 978,789 times since Tuesday

D) Don't

E) Fucking

Grumpy & Me

F) Do

G) It

H) Hire a professional...hitman or decorator. Either will suffice.

I really dislike Grumpy intensely after a few days locked in the same room. I came to this conclusion when he actually quizzed me on my poor application of wallpaper paste. I pasted his arse when he was up the ladder and asked if it was thick enough. He replied that it would take a lot more paste to match my rhinocerarse.

Z) Don't fucking do it......ever.....

We're Going on a Sofa Hunt

WE WERE LIKE the three bears, minus one, on yesterday's sofa hunt.

This one is too hard. This one is too soft. Too high. Too low. Too slippery. Too squishy. Too long. Too short.

"It's trying to eat my arse."

"It's the wrong shade of brown."

"Eeww."

"You are fucking joking."

After we sat on seventy-hundred and ten, we retired for cake. How the hell is sitting down so tiring?

Grumpy had to reenact his *reading paper* position. his *drinking tea* position, and his *correcting the world leaders on TV* position. Strangely, each position made him look like he was taking a shit. So I pretended I wasn't with him, except he kept talking to me. Loudly.

We realised what short little fuckers we are when

several sofas rejected us because our feet didn't touch the floor. We slid off one or two. And the one I thought I really liked nearly snapped my spine when I dropped onto it a bit too heavily.

The one I had seen several months earlier was reduced to half price. I still loved it. The problem is I quite like modern. Grumpy's choice is nursing home chic, complete with heavy patterns so any stains are camouflaged (reference "Eeww" above).

I completely lost him in the grandfather clock section. After retracing my steps, I found him hugging the biggest one with his head resting against it, so he could hear the ticking. It looked like a scene out of *The Revenant*.

Just before closing, Grumpy agreed I could pick the one I thought was best.

Last night, I tossed and turned all night. I had nightmares about fucking sofas. The bastards were chasing me all over the street. Fast-moving, big buggers on their well-oiled castors. Bulging feather-filled cushions threatening to suffocate me. Then the wide-awake questions after I refused to close my eyes and be chased again. Could you lie on the new one under a duvet when you were under the weather? Will

Grumpy wear a hole in the wooden arms? (Yes, he has made holes in the arms of sofas with his constant hand movements.) How will we get rid of the old one (which is still in good condition)? Do we really need a new sofa?

I never realised that old age meant so much procrastination, whether the question is to have cabbage for dinner, to have another pee before leaving the house, or buying something new.

Grumpy is busy measuring the lounge. Part of me hopes the new sofa is too big to fit. Sofa, so good.

An Ode to Fatty Bum Bum

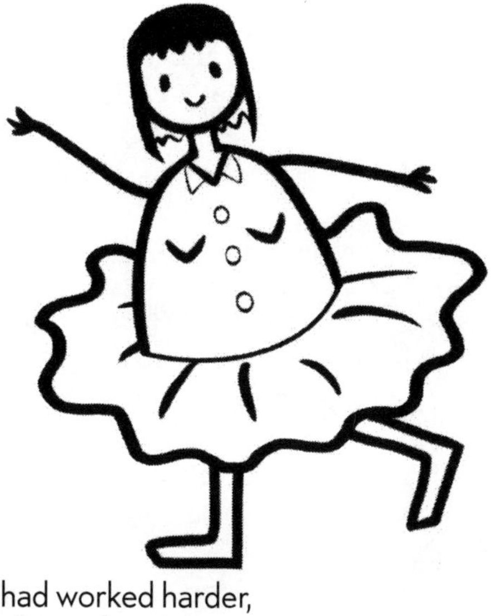

I wish I had worked harder,
And really tried my best,
And took the time to concentrate and never taken
rest.

I wish I could do handstands and twiddly, widdly swirls,
And flounce around in stiletto heels like many other girls.
I should have learned to shimmy,
And held my bosoms high,
And slapped on bright red lipstick; a girl should really try.
I often sit and wonder in this age of time to rest,
Is it too late to learn to pole dance, or am I really past my best?
So off I went and signed up and was given my own pole,
I kept it all a secret. I didn't tell a soul.
They made it look so easy; it soon would be my turn,
But as I grasped and try to lift, my face began to gurn.
My tits began to wobbly, my belly joined in too,
And all attempts to jump around just made me need the loo.
The lady was quite nice, and said it takes a lot of skill,
And could I give the floor a wipe where my pee had made a spill?
She said burlesque was gentler, and I should give that a try,
As she led me to the doorway and pushed me out:

Grumpy & Me

Goodbye.
I quite like all those feathers and tights, and heels et all,
I shall sign up for burlesque and have myself a ball.
I had the full big knickers and a sturdy bra to boot,
I would happily shake my tail feathers and simply have a hoot.
But when they said now take it off and shake them all about,
I had to stop and think a bit, 'tis not safe to let them out,
Because they cause a trip hazard and spread about the floor,
And that was when the fuckers pointed me to the door.
I cannot do the Can Can,
I am a lot more roll than rock,
Just thinking of the splits and my hips begin to lock.
I could be a ballerina and dance a dying swan,
But before I don a tutu, thirteen stone I would need gone.
It turns out physical exertion is clearly not for me,
As at the slightest jigging, I simply start to pee.
My tits are like a chariot and swing a-way down low,

And they threaten to abandon ship if up my arms I throw.
If I go into the downward dog, my arse begins to fart,
So I was asked to leave the yoga class because I made eyes smart.
Now when I ring the leisure centre or any local gym,
They say there are no vacancies, they cannot fit me in.
I shall have to accept in old age, I shall remain as fat,
And to be quite honest, I am quite okay with that.
So I'm off home to celebrate with tonic and with gin,
But I intend to sue Cadbury because without them, I'd be thin.

If you enjoyed book one of Grumpy & Me, please let me know. I've got lots more books in me, and I'd loved to share them with you!

Cheers,
Meg

Printed in Dunstable, United Kingdom

75178045R00136